Breast Imaging
Companion

Breast Imaging Companion

Gilda Cardenosa, MD

Head, Section of Breast Imaging
The Cleveland Clinic Foundation
9500 Euclid Avenue
Cleveland, Ohio

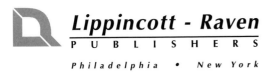

Lippincott - Raven
P U B L I S H E R S
Philadelphia • New York

Acquisitions Editor: James Ryan
Developmental Editor: Brian Brown
Project Editor: Patricia Connelly
Production Manager: Caren Erlichman
Production Coordinator: David Yurkovich
Design Coordinator: Doug Smock
Indexer: Wyman Indexing
Compositor: Maryland Composition
Printer: Quebecor-Kingsport

Library of Congress Cataloging-in-Publication Data

Cardenosa, Gilda.
  Breast imaging companion / Gilda Cardenosa.
      p.   cm.
  Includes bibliographical references and index.
  ISBN 0-397-51778-5
  1. Breast—Cancer—Diagnosis. 2. Breast—Imaging. I. Title.
  [DNLM: 1. Breast Neoplasms—radiography—handbooks.
  2. Mammography—handbooks.   WP 39 C266b 1997]
  RC280.B8C366   1997
  616.99′44907572—dc20
  DNLM/DLC
  for Library of Congress   96-29273
                                                                  CIP

Care has been taken to confirm the accuracy of the information presented and to describe generally accepted practices. However, the authors, editors, and publisher are not responsible for errors or omissions or for any consequences from application of the information in this book and make no warranty, express or implied, with respect to the contents of the publication.

The authors, editors, and publisher have exerted every effort to ensure that drug selection and dosage set forth in this text are in accordance with current recommendations and practice at the time of publication. However, in view of ongoing research, changes in government regulations, and the constant flow of information relating to drug therapy and drug reactions, the reader is urged to check the package insert for each drug for any change in indications and dosage and for added warnings and precautions. This is particularly important when the recommended agent is a new or infrequently employed drug.

Some drugs and medical devices presented in this publication have Food and Drug Administration (FDA) clearance for limited use in restricted research settings. It is the responsibility of the health care provider to ascertain the FDA status of each drug or device planned for use in their clinical practice.

9 8 7 6 5 4 3 2

To my parents
Gilda Paniza Cardeñosa and Ricardo Cardeñosa Barriga
and
Dr. Regina O'Brien

You've believed in me every step of the way
and in the journey, taught me much about perseverance and tenacity.
With you on my side, I've been able to soar in the face of adversity.
Thank you.

PREFACE

This book is targeted to radiology residents, however, it is my fervent hope that there is something (if only a few "pearls") here for anyone involved in breast imaging. Within the context of the prescribed format, I have tried to pack as much information as possible; even some of the figure legends introduce material. However, it should be clear that this is by no means an exhaustive review of breast imaging or an exhaustive review or discussion of the topics selected for presentation. It is my intention that this book serve as an introduction, overview, and review of breast imaging—a quick reference.

The material can be presented in many different ways. I recognize that my presentation and compartmentalization of the material is arbitrary; however, I want to emphasize the importance of having a working knowledge and understanding of clinical information, breast anatomy, and histology in addition to imaging related issues. As the role of the radiologist in the management of breast diseases continues to evolve, the ability to understand and correlate clinical, mammographic, ultrasonographic, and pathologic findings is increasing in importance.

Randomized controlled screening mammography trials have proven that the management of breast cancer, as we have known it, can be revolutionized (and has been in countries adhering to routine mass population screening programs). Breast cancer can be driven from the clinical presentation realm (advanced disease in many patients) to the mammographic/radiologic realm, as we strive to detect clinically occult, minimal cancers and save lives. As radiologists, we must acknowledge the role we can play. Recognizing and assuming the responsibilities that come with this role is the next necessary step.

We should emphasize the production of high-quality screening studies and complete thorough work-ups of women with screen detected possible abnormalities, and those presenting with clinical problems. We should expend resources in making our technologists and clerical personnel integral parts of the mammographic team. In interacting with women directly, their diligence, interest, and dedication to obtaining pertinent history and helping take care of our patients is extremely important in the success of any breast imaging facility and in the continued compliance, by patients, with our recommendations.

Our own interpretative abilities can be improved through ongoing continuing education and experience. Mammographic interpretation can be an extremely humbling experience. Every day brings a new lesson (sometimes one we thought we'd already learned). As we push the time of breast cancer diagnosis to earlier and earlier stages, we must be prepared to become an integral part of the therapeutic team. After all, the findings are radiologic and the diagnosis is now the purview of the radiologist. Familiar with his/her own medical audit results, the radiologist is the best equipped to communicate the significance of a particular finding to the patient and her referring physician. Thorough mammographic work-ups may yield information critical to the appropriate management of patients such as the presence of multicentric disease, bilateral breast cancer, and infiltrating ductal carcinomas with possible extensive intraductal components. After localizations, core biopsies, and specimen radiography, we need to communicate effectively with the surgeons, pathologists, and oncologists (radiation and medical).

Data keeping and tracking and an insistence on correlating mammographic and pathologic findings should also be the responsibility of the mammographer. These radiology–pathology correlation sessions are a great learning tool, effectively leading to improvements in a radiologist's interpretative abilities. Most importantly, however, if radiographic and pathologic findings are not congruent (and the radiologist may be the only one who can determine if there is radiology–pathology congruence), histologic reevaluation can be undertaken or if needed, the patient herself can be reexamined. In the end, the radiologist can be at the center of optimizing quality patient care.

Breast cancer, its heterogeneity, biology, and imaging, is a challenging and fascinating field of endeavor. Through our involvement and commitment, we can revolutionize breast cancer management in our communities—we can save lives, many lives. If, through this minor effort, I peak your interest or lure some of you into considering what can be an extremely rewarding specialty, I will reap the greatest reward of all.

ACKNOWLEDGMENTS

There is nothing I can say or write to adequately express my gratitude to Ms. Danette Doubet and Ms. Karol Burton, two extraordinarily talented and dedicated ladies who labored with me and kept me on course throughout this endeavor.

Sherry Aldridge, Mary Beecham, Tom Bortscheller, Sherry Brenneman, Joyce Davis, Jeff Doyle, Marsha Giacobazzi, Gaylen Greer, Gary Martin, Steve Masters, Joyce Oard, Jim Pesch, Don Phelps, and Philip Schleeter at the Caterpillar Image Lab, are an incredible group of people—every time I needed contact sheets, prints and/or diagrams done yesterday, (which was practically always) they came through with outstanding work. I appreciate and congratulate your commitment to excellence.

At Lippincott-Raven Publishers, Jim Ryan, Editor-in-Chief of Clinical Medicine and Brian Brown were invaluable in the development of this project. Mr. Ryan proposed and got the project off the ground and Mr. Brown, with an inordinate amount of patience, provided support and guidance. I would also like to thank Design Coordinator, Doug Smock, Production Manager, Caren Erlichman, Production Coordinator, David Yurkovich, and Project Editor, Pat Connelly. Your efforts were welcomed and appreciated greatly.

Dr. László Tabár's scientific contributions to breast imaging are far reaching. His challenges and thought provoking style make him an unrivaled *teacher*.

A special acknowledgment to Dr. G. W. Eklund, a superb *physician,* good friend, and colleague. We learned, thrived, and had fun in the process. This opportunity would not have come my way, if Dr. Eklund had not promoted me selflessly and actively, or if he had not created a wonderfully encouraging and challenging atmosphere at the Komen Breast Center. As you've written: "Thank you, dear friend."

Dr. Peter Dempsey, has supported and promoted me. His critical review of this book was wonderfully complete and helpful. Thank you for your encouragement.

The Sisters of the Third Order of Saint Francis have supported the Susan G. Komen Breast Center financially and spiritually from the beginning. As part of their mission in serving patients, the Sisters have provided the community with a warm and beautiful facility, equipped with the latest in technology and staffed with personnel dedicated to each of our patients. The *administrators* (Keith Steffen, Judy Shaheen, Judy Searle, Tori Badger, Ron Jost), *technologists* past and present (Dawn Brockhouse, Kathy Harrison, Trish Ingle, Pam Lee, Gail McCrabb, Rosemary McGraw, Amy Rammage, Heather Salzer, Vicki Shay,

Vicki Vornkahl-Thomas, Evelyn Walters, Tina Taggart, Connie Hodel, Janice Freeman, Mary Lascelles), *mammography assistants* (Cheryl Martin, Judy Schlosser) and *clerical staff* past and present (Marolyn Wakely, Debbie Carton, Diane Kneer, Gloria Warr, Peggy Irby, Nancy Brandstatter, Toby Bohm, Renae Douglas, Trudy Robinson, Kim Archdale, Beverly Knight) at the Komen Breast Center are some of the most dedicated individuals I have encountered in my career. Their professionalism and commitment shines on the Center and all of us who have been honored to work with them.

To the Peoria Community and in particular, our patients: your support of the breast cancer cause and your courage in fighting this disease is the major motivating factor for so many of us—you are the mission. Many thanks are also extended to the members of the Susan G. Komen Memorial Chapter of Peoria, Inc., who support and fund some of our clinical research endeavors at the Komen Breast Center.

Lastly, to many loyal friends and my parents who over the years have come to realize and accept that my job is a passion, second to none—and yet, support and cheer me through it all with unwavering love, thank you.

CONTENTS

Breast Imaging
Companion

Breast Imaging Companion
by Gilda Cardenosa
Lippincott-Raven Publishers, Philadelphia © 1997

Chapter 1

BREAST CANCER AND MAMMOGRAPHY: AN OVERVIEW

Breast Cancer

KEY FACTS

- Excluding skin cancers, breast cancer is the most frequently diagnosed malignancy (31% of all cancers detected) and the second leading cause of cancer mortality (17% of all cancer deaths) in women.
- In 1996, 184,300 new cases will be detected; 44,300 women will die of breast cancer.
- One in 8 women (12.5%) will be affected in their lifetime (arguably an epidemic).
- Relevant risk factors
  - Patient age (breast cancer incidence increases with advancing age)
  - Personal history of breast cancer
  - Prior breast biopsy with certain benign diagnoses (proliferative changes with atypia: atypical ductal hyperplasia; lobular neoplasia; juvenile papillomatosis)
  - Family history (first-degree relative)—more significant if there is more than one relative or if breast cancer is bilateral or occurs in a premenopausal patient
  - BRCA-1, BRCA-2 genes (account for 5% of all breast cancers)
- Other factors associated with breast cancer risk (implicated, not strong risk factors) include:
  - Early age at menarche, late age at menopause
  - Nulliparity, late age at first live birth
  - No breast feeding
  - Postmenopausal obesity
  - History of exposure to high-dose radiation
- An 8.1% decrease in breast cancer mortality was reported for 1989–1992 by the Surveillance, Epidemiology, and End Results (SEER) program. At least part of this can be attributed to screening mammography and early breast cancer detection.

Risk Marker Lesions

KEY FACTS

- Relative risk (RR) is the rate of cancer in women with a given condition or diagnosis divided by the rate of cancer in the reference population.
  - The reference population should be defined, as this alters the calculated RR.
  - Other factors that affect RR are the patient's age at the time of biopsy and the number of follow-up years.
- No increased risk
  - No proliferative disease
  - Apocrine change
  - Duct ectasia
  - Mild epithelial hyperplasia
  - Adenosis
- Slightly increased RR (1.5 to 2 ×)
  - Proliferative disease without atypia
  - Moderate/florid ductal hyperplasia
  - Papilloma
  - Sclerosing adenosis
- Moderately increased RR (4 to 5 ×)
  - Proliferative disease with atypia
  - Atypical ductal hyperplasia
  - Atypical lobular hyperplasia
- High relative risk (8 to 10 ×)
  - Atypical ductal hyperplasia and a positive family history (first-degree relative)
  - Lobular neoplasia (lobular carcinoma in situ)
  - Well-differentiated ductal carcinoma in situ
- Complex fibroadenomas (see Chap. 10)
  - 2.17 × in women with noncomplex fibroadenomas
  - 3.10 × in women with complex fibroadenomas
  - 3.72 × in women with complex fibroadenomas and a positive family history
  - 3.88 × in women with complex fibroadenomas and benign proliferative changes in surrounding stroma
- Lesions suggested by some investigators as possibly associated with an increased breast cancer risk but currently lacking the epidemiologic studies to prove or disprove the contention
  - Multiple papillomas
  - Radial scars or complex sclerosing lesions
  - Juvenile papillomatosis

Screening: General Comments

KEY FACTS

- Breast cancer is a heterogeneous disease.

- The cause(s) of breast cancer is unknown, so prevention is not currently an option.

- There are no data to support the notion that currently available treatments affect the overall breast cancer mortality rate significantly.

- There is debate as to whether breast cancer is systemic from the beginning or is localized to the breast for variable periods before becoming systemic.

- If cancer is systemic from inception, early detection through mammographic screening would have little benefit. However, if it is localized to the breast for variable periods, early detection might be the only effective way of dealing with this epidemic.

- Tabár's data from the two-county Swedish screening trial strongly support the contention that breast cancer is localized to the breast for a variable period of time before the development of systemic disease.
  - Under these circumstances, the time to diagnosis becomes critical: the earlier breast cancer is detected, the less likely it is to have become systemic.
  - Irrespective of tumor grade and nodal status, breast cancers less than 1 cm in size have a 12-year survival rate of approximately 95%.
  - Node-negative breast cancers less than 1.5 cm in size have a 12-year survival rate of approximately 94%.

- Although prevention of breast cancer is not an option and current treatments are not likely to affect mortality rates significantly, early breast cancer detection can affect overall breast cancer mortality rates significantly.
  - We must screen a sufficiently large portion of the population to see effects.
  - We must screen at appropriate intervals.

- With the use of mammography (the best method for detecting early breast cancers reliably), breast cancers are missed:
  - If the threshold for intervention is high (ie, if we wait until a lesion is obviously cancer before recommending biopsy)
  - If the screening intervals are too long.
  - It is generally accepted that breast cancers grow more quickly in premenopausal women, so we recommend annual screening mammograms in all women starting at age 40.

- Issues to consider in proving screening efficacy
  - Lead time bias—thorough screening can detect breast cancers at an earlier date but this doesn't change time of death.
  - Length bias—there is a disproportionate numbers of slower growing tumors (better prognosis) in screened population.
  - Selection bias—self-selected patients (volunteers) may have better outcomes regardless of screening (better compliance, increased awareness).

- Overdiagnosis bias—screening detects lesions of questionable significance (ie, well-differentiated DCIS) with respect to overall patient mortality.

- Survival by itself it insufficient to establish an alteration in the natural history (or mortality) of breast.

- Randomized controlled trials are needed with mortality as an end point to overcome described biases.

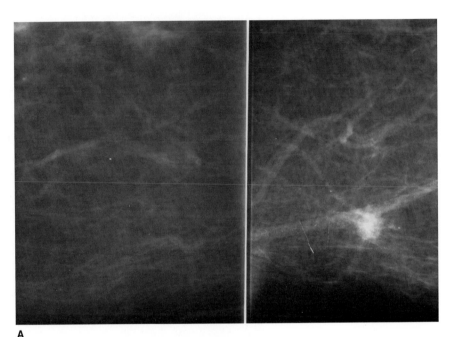

A

FIGURE 1-1   Poorly differentiated infiltrating ductal carcinoma. (**A**) Right craniocaudal views 1 year apart, back to back. A mass has developed in the medial portion of the breast. If screening mammography is to be effective, we must have appropriate thresholds for intervention and short enough screening intervals to detect developing lesions. We recommend annual screening mammography starting at age 40 for all women (and starting at age 30 for women with a family history of breast cancer).

(continued)

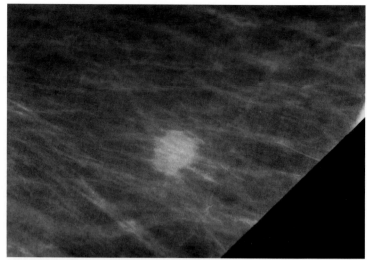

B

FIGURE 1-1 (CONTINUED)
(**B**) Spot magnification view demonstrating ill-defined margins of mass. (**C**) Solid, round mass on ultrasound (*arrow*). Solid, developing mass (neodensity) in postmenopausal patient not on estrogen requires biopsy.

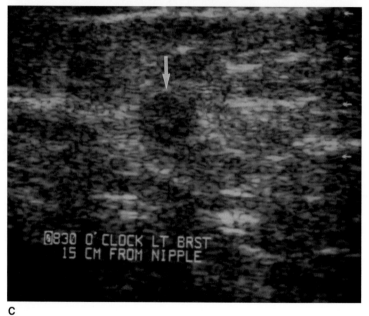

C

Screening Trials

KEY FACTS

- Randomized controlled trials are needed to prove the efficacy of screening.
  - Such trials must enroll enough women to have sufficient statistical power to prove a benefit from screening (ie, enough women must die in the control group to prove that the deaths do not occur in the study group). The smaller the difference (benefit) one is trying to prove, the larger the number of women needed to prove that difference.
  - Randomization should be blinded.
  - Technology, interpretation, and management of findings should be optimal and standardized.
  - Several randomized controlled trials of women starting at age 40 have shown 20% to 40% reductions in breast cancer mortality in the screened groups compared to controls.
  - Sufficient follow-up to see benefit is needed; in 40- to 49-year-old women, 10 to 15 years of follow-up are needed before screening benefit is seen.
  - It is generally accepted that screening mammography in women over age 50 is beneficial (ie, fewer women will die of breast cancer in the screened population). How logical is it to say that mammography does not work in women under age 50? What is magical about age 50? What happens to breast tissue when it is 50 years old?
  - Although there is some loss of breast tissue perimenopausally, one cannot predict patient age based on parenchymal patterns: young women may have fatty replaced breasts; older women may have dense tissue.
- Canadian National Breast Cancer Screening Trial
  - Only randomized controlled trial intended to evaluate screening benefit in 40- to 49-year-old women
  - Significant flaws in design and execution of trial
  - One-tenth the number of women needed to prove benefit enrolled in trial (50,000 women as opposed to 500,000 needed to prove benefit)
  - Problems with mammographic quality
  - Problems with randomization: more women with advanced lymph node-positive disease were randomized to the study group (women were examined by trained nurse-practitioners before randomization)
  - Lesion management protocols not standardized (some clinically occult lesions may not have been biopsied)

Screening Recommendations

- American Cancer Society
    - Baseline age 35 to 40
    - Mammography every 1 or 2 years in 40- to 49-year-old women
    - Annual mammography in women over age 50
    - Monthly breast self-examination
    - Annual physical examination by health-care provider
- If the woman is in a high-risk category, screening is started 10 years earlier (age 30), unless the mother's breast cancer occurred at an early age (before age 40), in which case we start 10 years before the age of detection (ie, if cancer detected at age 34 in mother, we start screening daughter at age 24).
- Women below age 30 who are pregnant or lactating and who present with clinical symptoms
    - Our starting point is correlative physical examination and ultrasound. A single mediolateral oblique view is sometimes done after the ultrasound.
    - We do not hesitate to do a complete mammogram if there is any question of an underlying malignancy.
- Young girls (8 to 12 years) presenting with a subareolar mass
    - Usually represents breast bud development
    - May be asymmetric but eventually becomes symmetric
    - Failure of breast development results if a biopsy is undertaken at this time (effectively, the breast bud is removed at the time of surgery).

Approach to Screening Mammograms

KEY FACTS

- Review images in a consistent manner every time, using high-luminance view-boxes (3500 NIT), with a mechanism to mask extraneous light.

- The only light in the reading room should come through the mammographic images. Extraneous light causes constriction of pupils, decreasing sensitivity to available light. With no ambient light, the observer's eyes become more efficient at gathering light coming through images.

- Craniocaudal (CC) views back to back; mediolateral oblique (MLO) views back to back; comparison studies (see below) over current CC and MLO views

- Images should be evaluated for technical factors. Do not settle for suboptimal quality. If you find yourself making excuses for the images, don't interpret—repeat!
    - Positioning: has all breast tissue been evaluated in two projections?
    - Is compression adequate? Is there motion or blur?
    - Contrast
    - Exposure

- Images should be viewed at a distance (facilitates appreciation of diffuse changes) and close up with a magnification lens.

- Specific areas to evaluate
    - Subareolar area
    - Retroglandular area in CC and MLO views
    - Medial aspect of breasts on CC views
    - On MLO views, superior cone of tissue
    - Glandular tissue/subcutaneous fat juncture

- You may want to evaluate the mammogram in parts in a systematic, consistent manner. The areas not being evaluated can be masked—evaluate lateral, middle, and medial portions on CC views and upper, middle, and inferior portions on MLO views. This approach focuses your attention on smaller segments of the breasts. Commercially available viewers can facilitate this process; these can come with built-in magnification.

- Comparison studies
    - Consider looking at studies that precede the current study by 2 or more years.
    - Subtle changes may not be apparent readily from 1 year to the next, but they become apparent when comparison is made to the earliest studies available.

- Do not be seduced by stability. If you see malignant calcifications or a spiculated mass (with no history of surgery or trauma or ongoing infection) today, recommend biopsy, even if the lesion has been stable for 1 or several years.

(text continues on the next page)

Approach to Screening Mammograms
(Continued)

- If there is an obvious lesion (clinical or mammographic), look away from it. Make sure you evaluate the remaining breast tissue and the contralateral breast before evaluating the obvious lesion. Do not let yourself be distracted!

- Double-reading screening mammograms (two readers evaluating screening studies independently) may increase the number of screen-detected cancers (6% to 15% increase in cancer detection reported with double-reading without increases in callback or biopsy recommendation rates).

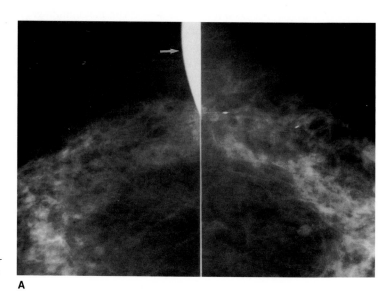

FIGURE 1-2
(A) Lesion exclusion. Right and left craniocaudal (CC) views. Breast tissue to edge of film laterally. How much tissue has been excluded and what might you be missing? Note patient-related artifact laterally on right CC view (*arrow*).

A

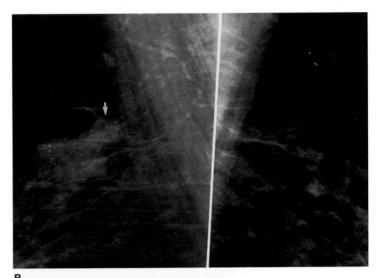

B

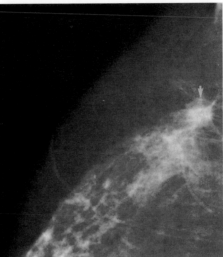

C

FIGURE 1-2 (CONTINUED)
(**B**) Right and left mediolateral oblique (MLO) views. Did you find the cancer? Asymmetric tissue on the right just anterior to the pectoral muscle margin (*arrow*). Are you skeptical? How would you dictate this? (**C**) Right exaggerated CC view. Spiculated mass at glandular/fat interface (*arrow*). In this projection we can see retroglandular fat. This lesion was excluded from the field of view on the routine CC view and was subtle on the MLO view—would you have detected it? With the exaggerated CC view it is readily apparent. Every effort should be made to see all breast tissue in two projections.

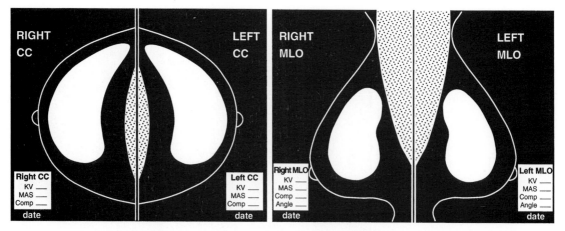

FIGURE 1-3   Diagram of screening mammogram. Right and left craniocaudal (CC) views back to back. By convention, metallic labels indicating view type are placed closest to axilla (on CC views laterally, on mediolateral oblique [MLO] views superiorly). Pectoral muscle is seen in 20% to 40% of all CC views; if the pectoral muscle is not seen, look for cleavage. Retroglandular fat is seen laterally, ensuring that all lateral tissue has been imaged. Right and left MLO views. Pectoral muscle to the level of the nipple and with convex anterior margin; the breast is pulled out and lifted up so that the inframammary fold is opened and a small amount of abdomen is included in the field of view. Labels, either attached to film or flashed onto film (along with patient's name and age, institution name, and date of study), should indicate kV, mAs, compression (in cm), and, for oblique view, the degree of obliquity so as to be able to troubleshoot (exposure, contrast, and blurring) effectively. Corresponding comparison films would be hung above current films.

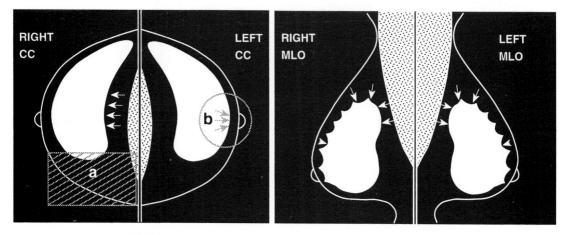

FIGURE 1-4   In addition to looking for microcalcifications, masses, and areas of architectural distortion specifically, it is important to assess the medial portion of the breasts on the CC view (*a*), the subareolar area on craniocaudal (CC) and mediolateral oblique (MLO) views (*b*), the glandular/fat interfaces on CC and MLO views (particularly the superior cone of tissue on the MLO view [*arrows*]), and the usually fatty area between the pectoral muscle and glandular tissue on the MLO view.

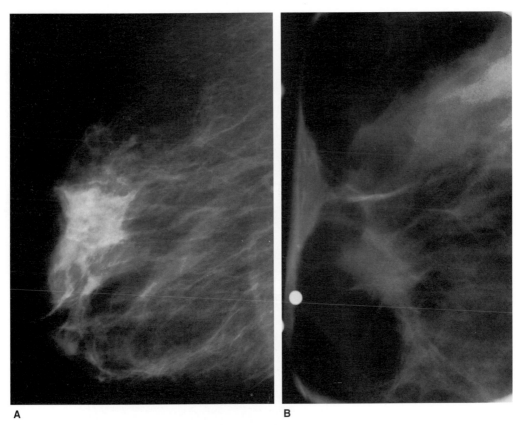

A   B

FIGURE 1-5 (A) Right mediolateral oblique (MLO) view. Can you find the cancer? Evaluate the subareolar area carefully. The subareolar area may be undercompressed (the base of the breast is thicker and may limit compression anteriorly) and is a ''busy'' area (confluence of ducts and nipple). Specifically evaluate the subareolar area. If there is any question of undercompression or blur, get an anterior compression (full paddle) view or spot compression of the subareolar area. (B) Infiltrating lobular carcinoma. Spot compression view, right subareolar area. Spiculated mass.

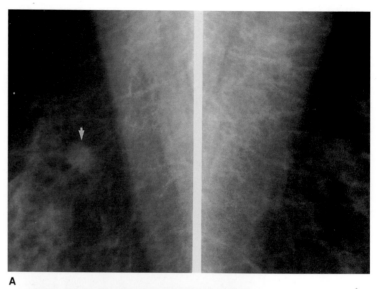

A

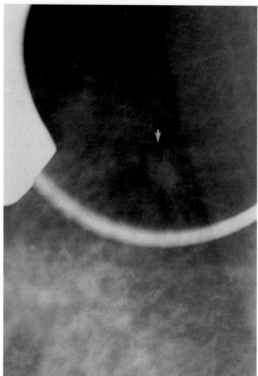

FIGURE 1-6
Infiltrating ductal carcinoma. (**A**)
Right and left mediolateral oblique
(MLO) views. Density on right MLO
view in fatty area between the pectoral muscle and glandular tissue
(*arrow*). Always evaluate this area.
Any asymmetry or nodule in this
area should cause you to consider the
possibilities. How would you handle
this? (**B**) Right MLO spot compression view. Spiculated mass is confirmed on the spot compression view.   B

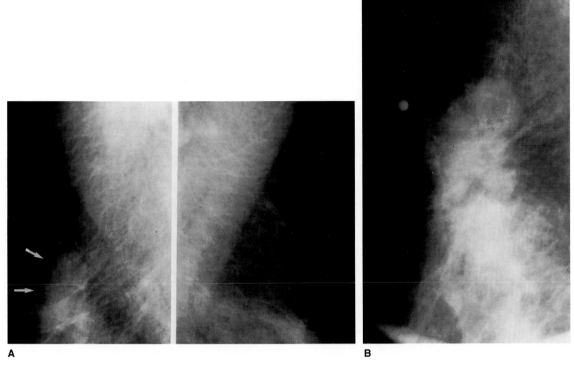

A   **B**

FIGURE 1-7   Infiltrating ductal carcinoma. (**A**) Right and left mediolateral oblique
(MLO) views. Asymmetric tissue (*arrows*) extending superiorly on the
right. Is this just normal asymmetric glandular tissue? How can you de-
cide? (**B**) Spot magnification views confirm the presence of a spiculated
mass with minimal skin retraction and thickening. This is not normal asymmetric glandular tissue.

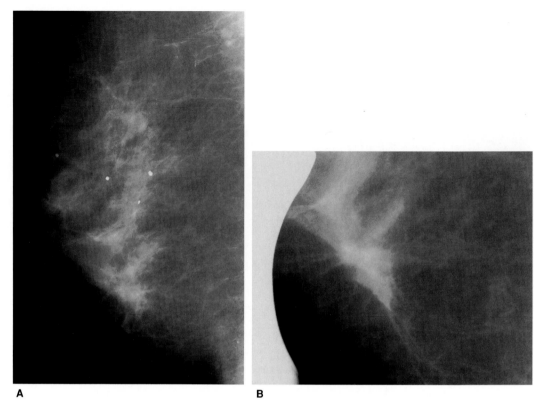

A   B

FIGURE 1-8   Infiltrating ductal carcinoma. (**A**) Did you find the cancer? Remember to evaluate the glandular tissue/fat interface: do you see distortion or a bulging contour? (**B**) Right oblique spot inferiorly, confirming spiculation and architectural distortion.

Looking For ...

KEY FACTS

- Screening is for asymptomatic women and entails two views of each breast (CC and MLO). In a few women, an exaggerated craniocaudal view may need to be done to evaluate lateral tissue in two projections.

- Screening views are for detection, not characterization or diagnosis. The decision algorithm on screening studies is simple: either normal or possibly abnormal (additional studies indicated).

- Diagnostic studies are done in women with abnormal screening studies (callbacks from screening) or in women with symptoms for further evaluation and characterization of the lesion.
    - Recommendation decisions can be simplified with additional views, ultrasound studies, and correlative physical examination.
    - We can provide information with respect to additional lesions (multicentricity), extent of disease, invasive disease with an associated extensive intraductal component, and so forth, if the lesion has been evaluated completely.

- Indications for diagnostic studies
    - Mass or masses (screen-detected or palpable)
    - Microcalcifications (usually screen-detected)
    - Architectural distortion (usually screen-detected but some are palpable)
    - Parenchymal asymmetry (usually screen-detected but some are palpable)
    - Palpable abnormality described by patient or referring physician
    - Focal tenderness
    - Spontaneous nipple discharge
    - Miscellaneous

- Be particularly careful with:
    - A neodensity in a postmenopausal women (particularly if not on estrogen)
    - Solid masses increasing in size
    - Increasing size or density at a postoperative site (it is also worth knowing the histology of the original biopsy)

Probably Benign Lesions

KEY FACTS

- Localized findings
    - Cluster of small, round or oval calcifications
    - Regardless of lesion size and patient age: nonpalpable, noncalcified, solid, round or oval, well-circumscribed mass (may have gentle lobulation); margins must be seen completely (ie, not obscured by surrounding breast tissue)
    - Nonpalpable, focal asymmetry with concave margins and interspersed fat
    - Asymptomatic (no nipple discharge), single dilated duct

- Multiple (three or more), similar findings, distributed randomly, often bilaterally
    - Circumscribed masses
    - Round or oval, small calcifications in tight clusters (or scattered individually throughout both breasts)

- If after appropriate evaluation (diagnostic work-up, including additional views and ultrasound), a lesion meets the above criteria, periodic mammographic follow-up can be undertaken. These lesions do not need to be biopsied unless:
    - The woman is extremely anxious and follow-up will affect her quality of life
    - The woman is unlikely to return for follow-up (poor compliance)
    - The woman is pregnant or planning pregnancy

- The likelihood of malignancy is low for probably benign lesions (1.4% reported by Sickles).

- Probably benign masses that are actually malignant can be detected with changes on follow-up studies.
    - Prognostically, the size, nodal status, and clinical course of these lesions when detected (after follow-up studies) are reportedly no different from those of malignancies diagnosed at the time of initial screening.

- Follow-up, when recommended, is usually a 6-month follow-up to be repeated four to six times (two examinations of the affected breast yearly for 2 to 3 years).
    - Three-month follow-ups should not be done on a routine basis. The only indication for 3- or 4-month follow-ups is in evaluating postsurgical changes or inflammatory conditions, situations in which one expects to see a rapid change.
    - Short-term follow-ups are intended for probably benign lesions. If you are expecting a rapid change (ie, in 3 months), you should probably be considering biopsy today.

- Ultrasound characteristics
    - Hyperechogenicity
    - Ellipsoid
    - Gentle bi- or trilobed
    - Thin echogenic pseudocapsule

Malignant Characteristics

KEY FACTS

- Physical examination findings
  - Hard, gritty mass; little mobility
  - Tissue consistency difference (particularly if correlated with parenchymal asymmetry mammographically)
  - Skin thickening, retraction (dimpling), stretching, erythema, ulceration
- Mammography: mass
  - Spiculation (no history of previous surgery or trauma)
  - Ill-defined, microlobulation
  - Mass with malignant-type microcalcifications
  - Skin thickening, retraction
- Mammography: architectural distortion (no history of previous surgery or trauma)
- Mammography: microcalcifications
  - Linear, branching, casting calcifications
  - Pleomorphism
  - Multiple clusters
- Ultrasound
  - Marked hypoechogenicity
  - Spiculation
  - Angular margins
  - ''Taller than wide''
  - Shadowing
  - Branch pattern
  - Duct extension

Breast Cancer Staging (TNM Classification)

KEY FACTS

- Primary tumor
  - TX: primary tumor cannot be assessed
  - T0: no evidence of primary tumor
  - Tis: carcinoma in situ (ductal, lobular, or Paget's disease)
  - T1: greatest tumor dimension 2 cm or less
  - T1a: greatest tumor dimension 0.5 cm
  - T1b: greatest tumor dimension 0.5 to 1 cm
  - T1c: greatest tumor dimension 1 to 2 cm
  - T2: greatest tumor dimension 2 to 5 cm
  - T3: greatest tumor dimension more than 5 cm
  - T4: any-sized tumor with extension to chest wall
  - T4a: chest wall extension
  - T4b: breast skin edema or ulceration
  - T4c: both T4a and T4b
  - T4d: inflammatory carcinoma
- Regional lymph nodes (pathologic—pN)
  - pNX: regional nodes cannot be assessed
  - pN0: no regional node metastasis
  - pN1: metastases to movable ipsilateral lymph nodes
  - pN1a: micrometastases
  - pN1b: metastases larger than 0.2 cm
  - pN1bi: metastases to one to three nodes 0.2 to 2 cm
  - pN1bii: metastases to four or more nodes 0.2 to 2 cm
  - pN1biii: extension beyond node capsule; metastasis less than 2 cm
  - pN1biv: metastasis larger than 2 cm
  - pN2: metastasis to axillary nodes fixed to each other or to other structures
  - pN3: metastasis to ipsilateral internal mammary
- Distant metastasis
  - MX: presence of distant metastasis cannot be assessed
  - M0: no distant metastasis
  - M1: distant metastasis present

From American Joint Committee on Cancer (AJCC) and International Union Against Cancer (UICC), 1992.

Breast Cancer Staging (Stages)

KEY FACTS

- Stage 0
  - Tis N0, M0
- Stage I
  - T1 N0 M0
- Stage IIA
  - T0 N1 M0
  - T1 N1 M0
  - T2 N0 M0
- Stage IIB
  - T2 N1 M0
  - T3 N0 M0
- Stage IIIA
  - T0 N2 M0
  - T1 N2 M0
  - T2 N2 M0
  - T3 N1 M0
  - T3 N2 M0
- Stage IIIB
  - T4 any N M0
  - Any T N3 M0
- Stage IV
  - Any T any N M1

From American Joint Committee on Cancer (AJCC) and International Union Against Cancer (UICC), 1992.

BIBLIOGRAPHY

Bird RE. Screening mammography: approach to interpretation and value of double reading. RSNA Categorical Course in Breast Imaging Syllabus 1995, pp 73–76

Cardenosa G, Eklund GW. Screening mammography in women 40–49 years old. AJR 1995; 164:1104–1106

Dupont WD, Page DL, Parl FF, et al. Long-term risk of breast cancer in women with fibroadenoma. N Engl J Med 1994;331:10–15

Kopans DB, Feig SA. The Canadian National Breast Screening Study: a critical review. AJR 1993;161:755–760

Moskowitz M. Breast cancer: age-specific growth rates and screening strategies. Radiology 1986;161:37–41

Page DL, Dupont WD. Premalignant conditions and markers of elevated risk in the breast and their management. Surg Clin North Am 1990;70:831–851

Sickles EA. Periodic mammographic follow-up of probably benign lesions: results in 3,184 consecutive cases. Radiology 1991;179:463–468

Sickles EA. Nonpalpable, circumscribed, noncalcified solid breast masses: likelihood of malignancy based on lesion size and age of patient. Radiology 1994;192:439–442

Sickles EA. Management of probably benign lesions. RSNA Categorical Course in Breast Imaging Syllabus 1995, pp 133–138

Smith RA. The epidemiology of breast cancer. RSNA Categorical Course in Breast Imaging Syllabus 1995, pp 7–20

Tabár L, Dean PB. Teaching atlas of mammography. New York: Thieme Verlag, 1985

Tabár L, Duffy SW, Warren Burhenne L. New Swedish breast cancer detection results for women aged 40–49. Cancer 1993;72(suppl):1437–1448

Tabár L, Fagerberg G, Day NE, Duffy SW, Kitchin RM. Breast cancer treatment and natural history: new insights from result of screening. Lancet 1992;1:412–414

Tabár L, Faberberg G, Duffy SW, Day NE, Gad A, Grontoft O. Update of the Swedish two-county program of mammographic screening for breast cancer. Radiol Clin North Am 1992;30:187–210

Varas X, Leborgne F, Leborgne JH. Nonpalpable, probably benign lesions: role of follow-up mammography. Radiology 1992;184:409–414

Breast Imaging Companion
by Gilda Cardenosa
Lippincott-Raven Publishers, Philadelphia © 1997

Chapter 2

QUALITY CONTROL

American College of Radiology (ACR) Mammography Accreditation Program

KEY FACTS

- 1985: Nationwide Evaluation of X-Ray Trends (NEXT 85)
  - Radiation dose and image quality at 232 U.S. mammography sites
  - Wide variation in image quality and radiation dose
- 1986: Galkin and associates survey 26 mammography sites in Philadelphia area
  - Tenfold range in average glandular doses
  - Site-to-site variation in image quality
  - Wide variations in film processor performance over 15-day period in 41% of facilities
- Concurrently, the American Cancer Society (ACS), through its National Breast Cancer Awareness screening programs, wanted to encourage mammographic screening nationally.
  - How to ensure high-quality mammograms at low radiation doses?
  - ACR approached by ACS about accreditation program.
- 1986: ACR designs and pilots mammography equipment testing program
- August 1987: accreditation of sites by ACR begins
  - Voluntary program
- Goals of ACR accreditation program
  - Establish quality standards for mammography
  - Mechanism for mammography sites to compare themselves with nationwide standards
  - Collection and dissemination of data on mammography practices
  - Encourage quality assurance
  - Reproducible, high-quality images at low radiation dose to patient
- ACR Mammography Accreditation Program: five components submitted by applicant
  - Site survey questionnaire
  - Phantom assessment of image quality
  - Dosimeter assessment of average glandular dose
  - Assessment of clinical images (submit mammograms one each of fatty and dense breasts)
  - Assessment of processor performance

Mammography Quality Standards Act of 1992

KEY FACTS

- Mammography Quality Standards Act (MQSA) of 1992 requires all mammography facilities (except those of the Department of Veterans Affairs) in the United States to be certified by the Food and Drug Administration starting October 1, 1994.

- Standards for personnel (interpreting physicians, technologists, physicists), equipment, maximum allowable dose, quality assurance, medical audit, outcome analysis, and record keeping and reporting

- Mammography facilities must apply and become accredited by an FDA-approved accreditation body: ACR, states of Iowa, California, and Arkansas are currently FDA-approved accrediting bodies.

- Facilities to be inspected annually by MQSA inspectors
  - Equipment performance (image quality and dose)
  - Quality assurance records
  - Quality control records and tests (technologists' tests and annual physicist report)
  - Medical audit and outcome analysis records
  - Mammography reports and films
  - Personnel qualification records

- Level 1 noncompliance (requires immediate action to remedy; reinspection and sanctions if corrective action is not undertaken)
  - Program for high-quality mammography not fully instituted
  - Unqualified personnel
  - Nondedicated mammography equipment
  - Radiation dose 400 mrad/exposure or more

- Level 2 noncompliance (written response with corrective action required within 30 days of inspection)
  - Medical audit system lacking
  - Radiation dose 300 to 400 mrad/exposure
  - Phantom image fails minimum criteria

- Level 3 noncompliance (corrective action before next inspection)
  - Minor equipment problem or problems
  - All quality control tests not completed

- Federal Register publications of December 21, 1993 (MQSA interim rules), September 30, 1994 (amendments), and April 3, 1996 (proposed final rules)—Department of Health and Human Services; FDA

Quality Control Tests (Technologist)

- Daily
    - Darkroom cleanliness
    - Processor quality control
- Weekly
    - Screen cleanliness
    - Viewboxes and viewing conditions
- Monthly
    - Phantom images
    - Visual checklist
- Quarterly
    - Repeat analysis
    - Analysis of fixer retention in film
- Semiannually
    - Darkroom fog
    - Screen/film contact
    - Compression
- For each test, need to know:
    - Objective
    - Frequency
    - Equipment needed
    - Procedure
    - Any caveats
    - Performance criteria (corrective actions)
- Consult the ACR's *Mammography quality control manuals for medical physicists, physicians and technologists* for further details on the technologist's and physicist's quality control tests. Familiarity with these tests is important in troubleshooting technically suboptimal films.

Darkroom Cleanliness

- Objective
  - To minimize film artifact
- Frequency
  - Daily test
  - Before any films are processed for the day
- Equipment
  - Mop and pail
  - Lint-free towels
  - Liquid hand soap
- Procedure
  - Processor power and water ''on''
  - Darkroom floor: damp mop
  - Countertops cleared
  - Lint-free, clean, damp towel to wipe processor feed tray and countertops
  - Keep hands clean.
  - Wipe or vacuum overhead vents and safelights weekly before cleaning feed tray and countertops.
- Performance
  - Dust artifacts on films
- Darkroom general principles
  - Dust and dirt must be minimized: smoking, drinking, or eating is not permitted at any time.
  - Counter for loading and unloading cassettes should be clear of any objects (they collect dust).
  - There should be no overlying shelves (dust settles and collects on items placed on shelves above counters).
  - Darkroom ceiling should be made of solid material; tiles collect dust.
  - Heating and air conditioning ducts should not be placed over countertops.
  - Electrostatic air cleaners can be used to reduce dust and dirt.
  - Minimize static by maintaining darkroom humidity between 40% and 60% year-round. Materials that reduce static electricity should be used for countertops, and static discharge systems to provide a continuous flow of ionized air (reduce static) should also be used.

Processor Quality Control

- Objective
  - To verify that film processor chemicals are working in a consistent manner as specified by the manufacturer
- Frequency
  - At the beginning of each work day
- Equipment
  - Sensitometer (for single-emulsion film): 21 steps in 0.15 optical density increments
  - Densitometer
  - Fresh box of control film
  - Control chart
  - Thermometer (alcohol, dial, digital thermometer; do not use a mercury thermometer) accurate to at least 0.5°F
- Procedure: to establish operating levels for processor (new film, chemicals, or change in processing conditions)
  - Use a fresh box of film (reserve box of film for quality control).
  - Drain chemicals from processor, flush tanks and roller racks with water.
  - Drain replenisher tanks and refill with fresh replenisher.
  - Fill fixer tank with fixer solution.
  - Flush developer tank again with water.
  - Fill developer tank half full with developer, add specified amount of starter solution, and then add sufficient developer to fill developer tank.
  - Set developer temperature to within ±0.5°F specified by film manufacturer (underdeveloped films can result from lower developer temperatures, leading to decreased image contrast).
  - Set developer and fixer replenishment rates specified by film manufacturer.
  - After developer temperature has stabilized, check temperature with clinical fever thermometer.
  - Using sensitometer, expose and process sensitometric strip each day for 5 consecutive days.
  - As outlined below, the sensitometric strip should be processed in a consistent manner.
  - Using densitometer, read and record densities for each step (measure center of each step); also measure an area of processed film, not exposed.
  - Calculate 5-day average for each step.
  - Determine which step has average density closest to 1.20 mid-density (MD; speed point, speed index, speed step).
  - Determine which step is closest to 2.20 and which step is closest to 0.45: the difference between these steps is designated the density difference (DD).
  - The average density of the 5 days' unexposed areas is designated base plus fog (B + F).

Processor Quality Control

- Procedure: daily processor quality control
  - Before any patient films are done, expose and process sensitometric strip.
  - Processing of strips should be consistent from day to day.
    - Developer temperature should be as specified by manufacturer.
    - The less-exposed end of the strip should be inserted into the processor first.
    - The strip should be processed on the same side of the processor each time.
    - On single-emulsion film, the emulsion orientation should be the same.
    - Time between exposure and processing should be approximately the same each day.
  - Read density for three indicated steps and B + F.
  - Plot MD, DD, and B + F.
  - Determine if any point exceeds control limits.
  - Circle out-of-control points; determine and correct cause of the problem. Repeat test and note the cause of the problem in the "remarks" section of the control chart.
  - If trends develop, institute corrective action before obtaining an out-of-control data point.
- Caveats
  - Sensitometric strips should be processed and evaluated **before** processing clinical films.
  - Sensitometric strips should be processed within an hour of being exposed.
  - Calibrated densitometer must be used for reading strip; visual comparison is not adequate.
  - Developer temperature should be within 0.5°F of manufacturer-specified temperature.
  - Quality control must be carried out on sensitometer, densitometer, and thermometer.
  - No mercury-containing thermometer should be used in processor.
- Performance
  - Data points must be entered for every day of operation.
  - MD and DD should be within 0.10 of operating levels; if outside ±0.10 but within ±0.15, the test should be repeated. If value is confirmed, process clinical images but monitor processor closely.
  - If MD or DD exceeds ±0.15, identify and correct problem before processing any mammograms.
  - B + F should be within ±0.03; if it exceeds ±0.3, identify and correct problem before processing any mammograms.
  - Any corrective actions should be noted on chart.
  - Processor quality control charts should be retained for 1 year.
  - Sensitometric films quality control chart should be retained on a monthly basis.

Screen Cleanliness

- Objective
  - To ensure that mammographic screens and cassettes are free of dust and dirt particles
- Frequency
  - At least weekly
  - Depending on usage, screens and cassettes may need to be cleaned more often.
  - If any artifact is detected (because cassettes are numbered, repeated artifacts associated with a given cassette can be identified and corrected expeditiously)
- Equipment
  - Screen cleaner (screen manufacturer)
  - Lint-free gauze pad
  - Lint-free cloth
  - Camel's hair brush
  - Canned air
- Procedure
  - Clean screens using manufacturer's procedures and materials.
  - After cleaning with liquid cleaners, cassettes are stood up open and allowed to air dry.
- Caveats
  - Compressed air: need ''clean'' air (no moisture, oils, and so forth)
- Performance
  - Review clinical images—minus density artifacts should not be seen on a routine basis or associated with a specific cassette

Viewboxes and Viewing Conditions

- Objective
  - To optimize viewing conditions
  - Luminance of viewboxes, ambient room illumination, and light falling on viewboxes may affect interpretation.
  - Fluorescent tubes should be replaced every 18 to 24 months (brightness decreases with time). Replace all at one time: if one tube needs to be replaced (ie, flickering or burned out), then all should be replaced.
- Frequency
  - Weekly
- Equipment
  - Window cleaner
  - Towels
- Procedure
  - Clean viewbox surface, making sure all marks are removed.
  - Inspect viewboxes for luminance uniformity.
  - Ensure masking equipment functions properly.
  - Ensure there are no sources of bright light or reflection from viewbox surface in reading room.

Phantom Images

- Objective
  - To check that x-ray imaging system and film processor(s) are operating optimally with respect to film density, contrast (density difference), uniformity, and image quality
- Frequency
  - Initial: after equipment calibration and with fresh chemistry in processor
  - Monthly
  - After servicing any equipment
- Equipment
  - Mammographic phantom (4- to 4.5-cm-thick tissue equivalent breast phantom with fibers, specks, and masses)
  - The 4-mm-thick acrylic disc placed on phantom must be consistent in placement, and the disc should not obscure details in the phantom (disc can be attached to phantom permanently with Superglue).
  - Cassette and film
  - Original phantom and previous film
  - Control charts
  - Magnifying lens
- Procedure
  - Film from bin into cassette
  - Cassette in cassette holder
  - Phantom on cassette holder: edge of phantom aligned with chest wall side of image receptor
  - Compression device in contact with phantom
  - Phototimer: under center of wax insert (consistency in phototimer)
  - Manual: exposure time and mA selected
  - Expose: technical factors should be those commonly used for a 4.5-cm compressed breast
  - Exposure time or mAs plotted on control chart
  - Film processed in same processor used for mammographic films
  - Densities measured in area of disc and background, adjacent to disc (to the right or left of disc, perpendicular to anode—cathode axis)
  - Background density and density difference plotted (background density minus disc density)
  - Number of simulated fibers, speck groups, and masses visible on image determined
  - Image examined for nonuniform areas, artifacts (dirt, dust, grid- or processor-related), grid lines

- Caveats
  - Phantom images should be viewed by the same person, on the same viewbox, under the same viewing conditions, at the same time of day, using the magnifier (and viewboxes) used for clinical work.
  - If there is a problem, other tests are needed to determine which imaging chain component is causing the problem.
- Performance
  - Film density of 1.2 ± 0.20
  - $DD = 0.40 \pm 0.05$ (4-mm disc and 29 kVp)
  - Film densities should be similar among facilities and among units within a given facility.
  - mAs should not change by more than $\pm 15\%$.
  - The number of visualized objects (fibers, specks, and masses) should not change by more than 0.5. Minimum: four largest fibers, three largest speck groups, and three largest masses.
  - Retain phantom images for last full year.

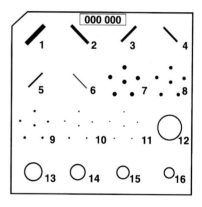

FIGURE 2-1
Details in RMI 156 phantom. Nylon fibers (1–6): 1.56, 1.12, 0.89, 0.75, 0.64, and 0.40 mm. Simulated microcalcifications (7–11): 0.54, 0.40, 0.32, 0.24, and 0.16 mm. Tumor-like mass (12–16): 2.00, 1.00, 0.75, 0.50, and 0.25 mm.

Visual Checklist

- Objective
  - To check that X-ray system indicator lights, displays, and mechanical locks and detents work properly
  - To ensure that the mechanical rigidity and stability of equipment is optimal
- Frequency
  - Monthly
  - After service, maintenance
- Equipment
  - Checklist
- Procedure
  - Review items on visual checklist
  - Date and initial
- Performance
  - All items in checklist should pass; if not, immediate corrective action should be taken.

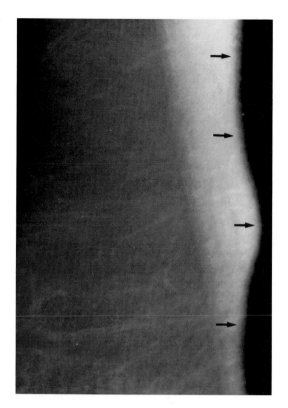

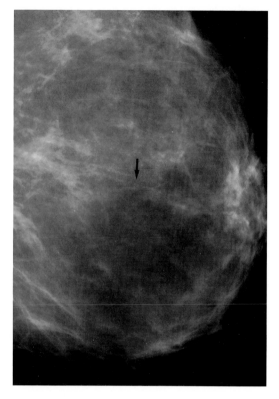

FIGURE 2-2
Film fog (*arrows*).

FIGURE 2-3
Film fog (*arrow*) resulting from a cracked safelight filter.

Screen/Film Contact

- Objective
  - To ensure optimal contact between film and screen
  - Resolution of mammography film is higher than that of conventional film (16 to 10 cycles/mm compared to 4 to 8 cycles/mm), so image sharpness can be significantly affected if there is poor film/screen contact.

- Frequency
  - Initially
  - For new screens
  - Semiannually
  - With reduced image sharpness

- Equipment
  - Copper screens (40 mesh or 40 wires per inch)
  - Acrylic sheets
  - Film
  - Densitometer (aperture 2.0 mm)
  - Screens and cassettes

- Procedure to be done for all cassettes
  - Clean screens and cassette.
  - Air dry cassettes for at least 30 minutes.
  - Load film in cassette (cassettes should have unique identifier number seen on images taken).
  - Wait 15 minutes.
  - Place cassette on top of cassette holder (no grid).
  - Place copper screen on top of cassette.
  - Place acrylic sheet or sheets (used to ensure exposure time will be at least 0.5 second) on top of compression device.
  - Move compression paddle (with acrylic sheets) as close to x-ray tube as possible (effectively reducing scatter radiation).
  - Select manual technique (25 to 28 kVp); film density should be 0.7 to 0.8.
  - Expose and process film.
  - Standing 3 feet away, view films on viewbox. Check for darker areas in mesh image.

- Performance
  - Areas of poor contact larger than 1 cm not eliminated by recleaning cassette are unacceptable.
  - Five or more areas less than 1 cm are acceptable; cassettes can be used.

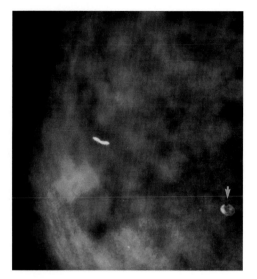

FIGURE 2-4
Poor film/screen contact. Artifact on screen (high density in center) precludes good film/screen contact focally—film is lifted off the screen by the artifact. Blur surrounding artifact. Benign lucent centered calcification (*arrow*).

Compression

- Objective
  - To ensure adequate compression in manual and powered modes.
- Frequency
  - Initially
  - Semiannually
  - When problems with compression adequacy are suspected
- Equipment
  - Flat, analog-type bathroom scale
  - Towels
- Procedure
  - Place towel on cassette holder for protection.
  - Place bathroom scale on towel, with center of scale directly under compression paddle.
  - Place one or more towels on top of scale.
  - Allow power drive to operate compression until it stops automatically.
  - Read and record compression applied.
  - Release compression.
  - Use manual drive until compression paddle stops.
  - Read and record.
  - Release compression.
- Caveat
  - Compression paddle may be damaged if safety mechanism is not adjusted properly. If 40 pounds is exceeded in the power mode, immediately release compression and service unit for appropriate adjustments.
- Performance
  - Range of compression force: 25 to 40 lb with power mode, at least 25 lb with manual drive (forces in excess of 40 lb are acceptable)

Quality Control Tests (Physicist)

- All tests should be done at least once annually.
- Mammography unit assembly evaluation
  - Proper operation of locks, detents, angulation indicators, and mechanical support
- Collimation assessment
  - Collimator cone should not allow significant radiation beyond edges of image receptor.
- Evaluation of focal spot performance
  - Measurement of focal spot dimensions
  - Slit camera
  - High-contrast resolution pattern
  - At least 13 line pair per mm with bars parallel to anode–cathode axis
  - At least 11 line pair per mm with bars perpendicular to anode–cathode axis
- kVp accuracy and reproducibility
  - kVp should be $\pm 5\%$ of indicated kVp and reproducible (coefficient of variation of 0.02)
- Beam quality assessment (half value layer [HVL] measurement)
  - HVL with compression paddle in place equals kVp/100 + 0.03 (mm of aluminum) or more
- Automatic exposure control (AEC) system performance assessment
- Uniformity of screen speed
- Breast entrance exposure, average glandular dose, and AEC reproducibility
  - Average glandular dose to average breast (4.2 cm of compression) less than 3 mGy (0.3 rads) per view for film/screen image receptors
  - Average glandular dose less than 1 mGy per view for nongrid film/screen image receptors
  - Average glandular dose less than 3 mGy per view for grid film/screen imaging receptors
- Image quality evaluation
  - 1.2 optical density at phantom center
  - 0.40 ± 0.05 density difference for 4-mm-thick disc and film exposed at 28 kVp
- Artifact evaluation

BIBLIOGRAPHY

American College of Radiology. Mammography quality control manuals for medical physicists, physicians and technologists. American College of Radiology, 1994

Galkin BM, Feig SA, Muir HD. The technical quality of mammography in centers participating in a regional breast cancer awareness program. RadioGraphics 1988;8:133–145

Hendrick RE. Quality assurance in mammography. Radiol Clin North Am 1992;30:243–255

Breast Imaging Companion
by Gilda Cardenosa
Lippincott-Raven Publishers, Philadelphia © 1997

Chapter 3

POSITIONING AND PROBLEM SOLVING

General Comments

KEY FACTS

- Breast cancer size at the time of diagnosis is an important prognostic factor. Regardless of histologic grade, a 10-year survival rate of greater than 90% can be obtained if tumors 10 mm or smaller can be diagnosed consistently.

- High-quality mammography can demonstrate invasive lesions 10 mm or smaller as well as noninvasive breast cancer (ductal carcinoma in situ) presenting with microcalcifications.

- Breast positioning during mammography is critical. Excluding breast tissue from the field of view may eliminate the opportunity to diagnose an early, potentially curable breast cancer.

- Although metallic BBs are used to mark areas of clinical concern, every effort should be made to ensure that the BB is in the right area and that the lesion has not been excluded from the field of view during positioning. This is particularly applicable to lesions close to the chest wall.

- The inferior and lateral margins of the breast are mobile; the upper and medial portions of the breast are fixed in position. During mammographic positioning, natural breast mobility should be used to maximize the amount of tissue included in the images (to minimize breast tissue exclusion).

- Posterior nipple line (PNL)
  - If the mediolateral oblique (MLO) views are positioned appropriately (convex muscle border to nipple level), draw a line along the anterior margin of the pectoral muscle, drop a perpendicular line from nipple to muscle, and measure. This is the PNL. It is predicated on optimal MLO positioning.
  - On the craniocaudal (CC) view, measure from the nipple back to the edge of the film, regardless of whether you see pectoral muscle or not. The PNL measurement on the CC view should be within 1 cm of the measurement obtained on the respective MLO view. If it is not within 1 cm, tissue has been excluded on the CC view.

- In some women, additional views (eg, exaggerated CCs) may be needed to image all breast tissue in two projections. In addition to positioning, mammographic images must be evaluated for appropriate exposure, contrast, resolution, and compression.

- Depending on breast size, 18 × 24 cm (8 in × 10 in) or 24 × 30 cm (10 in × 12 in) cassettes are available. Women with large breasts may require more than two views of each breast to image all breast tissue. For the MLO views, you may need to image the upper portion of the breast in one view and the lower portion in a second view. Do whatever it takes to ensure all breast tissue is imaged in two different projections.

- For women with small breasts or the male breast, narrow compression paddles (approximately half the width of the regular compression paddle) are available for optimal positioning.

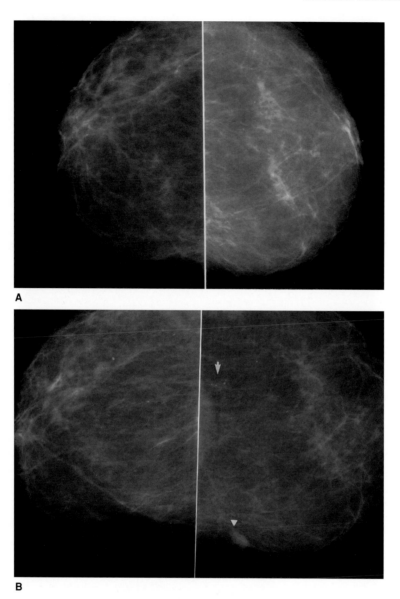

A

B

FIGURE 3-1   (A) Suboptimal positioning with resultant tissue exclusion. This study was accepted and interpreted. Actually, over 2 cm of tissue has been excluded from the field of view, including a cluster of calcifications posteriorly and a mass medially on the left. Remember to compare posterior nipple line measurements on mediolateral oblique and craniocaudal (CC) views. (B) Tissue visualization can be maximized with attention to positioning techniques. Right and left CC views with lifting of the inframammary fold and pulling of breast outwardly. Note calcifications (*arrow*) and mass medially on the left (*arrowhead*) not imaged on Figure 3-1A.

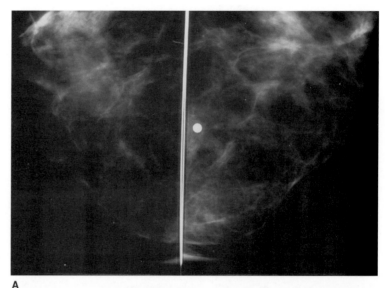

A

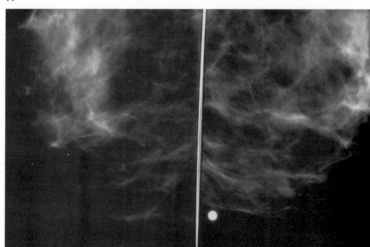

B

FIGURE 3-2

(**A**) Right and left craniocaudal views with metallic BB purportedly marking area of palpable mass. No abnormality is apparent in area of BB. (**B**) Right and left mediolateral oblique views with metallic BB placed over purported area of clinical concern. No abnormality is readily apparent. This is a relatively fatty area. (**C**) Hypoechoic mass corresponding to area of clinical concern. Given the posterior location of this lesion, the mass was actually not included in any of the mammographic views obtained. This underscores the importance of ensuring clinical correlation and lesion inclusion in the field of view. Ask yourself, has the area of clinical concern been included in the images? Is there any chance that because of lesion location or BB placement, the area of concern has been excluded? (The mass was a fibroadenoma on histology.)

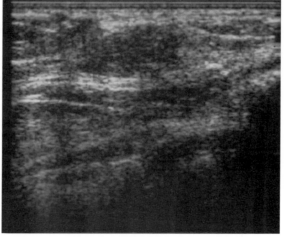

C

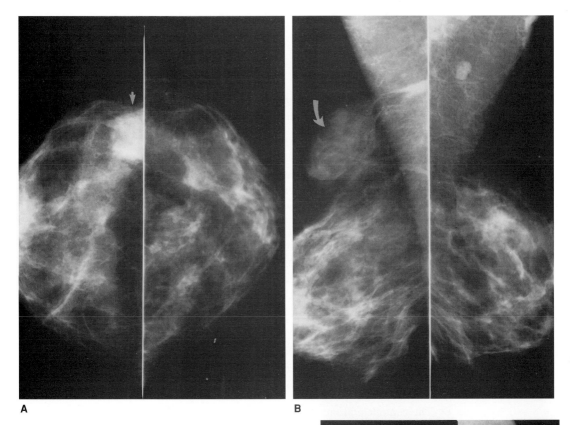

A   B

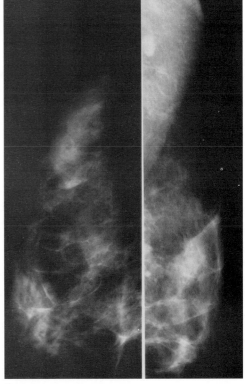

FIGURE 3-3
(**A**) Right and left craniocaudal (CC) views. An island of accessory tissue partially seen appears mass-like on the right laterally (*arrow*). On the left, retroglandular fat is seen laterally.
The mediolateral oblique (MLO) view should be reviewed for
confirmation of tissue (or a mass) extending superolaterally.
(**B**) Right and left MLO views. An oval area of glandular tissue (*arrow*) can be seen extending superiorly on the right. This
tissue has been evaluated incompletely in the CC projection.
On the left, as expected from the CC view, no tissue is seen on
the MLO extending superiorly. (**C**) Right and left exaggerated
CC views. Retroglandular fat is now seen on the right. With
the appearance of this area on MLO and exaggerated CC
views, what appears as a possible mass on the CC view is confirmed to be an island of accessory, normal glandular tissue on
the right. If doubts remain, spot compression views, correlative
physical examination, or an ultrasound can be done to confirm
this as normal glandular tissue.

C

Craniocaudal

KEY FACTS

- Natural breast mobility

    - The inframammary fold (IMF) is identified and the breast is lifted to the extent of its natural mobility.

    - Breast mobility varies. In some women, it is several centimeters, but in others it may be less than 1 cm.

    - After breast mobilization, the film holder is moved to the elevated IMF position (care should be taken not to go above the elevated IMF position, as this may exclude inferior, posterior lesions) and back to the chest wall.

- Every millimeter the breast is mobilized upward is a millimeter less that the compression paddle must come down over fixed (not inherently mobile) upper tissue, thereby minimizing the possibility of tissue exclusion and skin stretching. Much of the ''pain'' associated with mammography is probably related to skin stretching as compression is applied, rather than to compression itself.

- Outward pull

    - As the breast is mobilized superiorly, tissue is also pulled out away from the body as much as possible.

    - The technologist should work from the medial side of the patient.

- The contralateral breast should be lifted and placed on the corner of the bucky. If the technologist is not careful, the contralateral breast can be an impediment to the film holder going back all the way to the chest wall. By interposing itself between the film holder and the chest wall, the contralateral breast can lead to the exclusion of medial/posterior tissue.

- The medial half of the breast must be included on CC views; at the same time, as much lateral tissue as possible should be imaged. As the compression paddle is coming down, the medial half of the breast is stabilized while the lateral portion of the breast is pulled in (lateral pull).

- The lateral pull is usually enough to bring lateral tissue into view on routine CC views so that retroglandular fat is seen posterior to lateral tissue. In approximately 10% of women, tissue extends to the edge of the film laterally even after the lateral pull. Exaggerated CC views (uni- or bilateral) are needed in these women to image lateral tissue. The presence of lateral and posterior tissue can be confirmed on the MLO (tissue superimposed on pectoral muscle superiorly and posteriorly).

- A skin fold develops in the most posterior portion of the breast laterally in many patients after the lateral pull. This is an indication that a lateral pull was attempted. The technologist can eliminate some of these skin folds by interposing her index finger between the compression paddle and the breast and then rolling the finger out, along with the skin fold, from under the paddle posteriorly.

- Pectoral muscle should be seen in approximately 30% to 40% of CC views. When seen, it ensures that posterior tissue has not been excluded.

- If pectoral muscle is not seen, look for cleavage. This ensures that, at least medially, no tissue has been excluded.

- In some women a triangular, round, or wedge-shaped density is seen medially on CC views. This represents either the sternal attachment of an otherwise atrophied pectoral muscle or the sternalis muscle. The sternalis muscle usually has a round, mass-like appearance and is an uncommon variant in chest wall musculature (muscle extending from the infraclavicular region to the caudal aspect of the sternum); it is more common unilaterally.

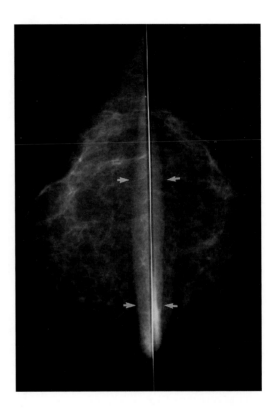

FIGURE 3-4
Right and left craniocaudal views. Pectoral muscle (*arrows*) is present bilaterally, confirming inclusion of posterior tissue. Laterally, retroglandular fat is seen.

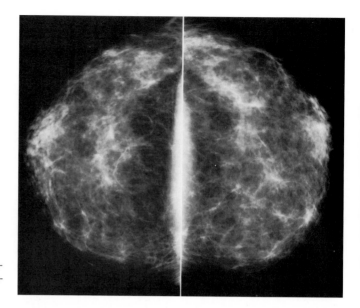

FIGURE 3-5
Right and left craniocaudal (CC) views. High-contrast, well-exposed CC views with visualization of the pectoral muscle bilaterally.

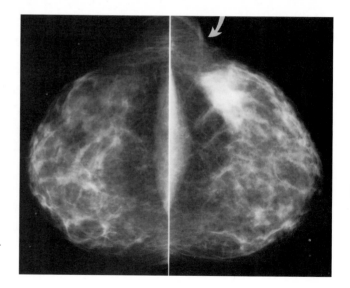

FIGURE 3-6
Right and left craniocaudal (CC) views. Retroglandular fat can be seen laterally. Skin fold (*arrow*) on the left laterally arises from the technologist doing lateral pull to include as much lateral tissue as possible on the CC view.

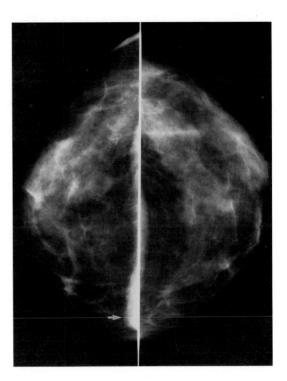

FIGURE 3-7
Right and left craniocaudal views. Rounded pectoral muscle medially on the right (*arrow*). This appearance is more commonly related to the sternal insertion of the pectoral muscle. When it is more focal and rounded, it may represent the sternalis muscle.

Mediolateral Oblique

KEY FACTS

- Natural breast mobility
  - The lateral portion of the breast is mobile and the medial portion is fixed.
  - The goal is to mobilize the lateral portion of the breast as much as possible to minimize medial tissue exclusion and skin stretching (medial half).
- Pectoral muscle relaxation
  - Mobilization of the breast and underlying pectoral muscle medially and outward pull of the breast tissue are facilitated if the pectoral muscle is relaxed.
  - As the pectoral muscle inserts on the upper portion of the humerus, the humeral head should be inwardly rotated, with the arm down behind the film holder or resting atop the film holder.
- Patient-specific angle of obliquity
  - The angle depends on the pectoral muscle orientation.
  - In maximizing the outward pull of a skin appendage (ie, the breast), it is best to pull parallel to underlying muscle fibers.
  - Depending on the woman's body habitus, the pectoral muscle has variable angles of obliquity. Short, stocky women have more horizontally oriented pectoral muscles; tall, thin women have more vertically oriented pectoral muscles.
- A small portion of the upper abdomen should be included, as breast tissue can extend to the IMF and below.
- The technologist should work from behind the patient. This allows the technologist to keep the patient from backing out of the unit even slightly.
  - From behind the patient, the technologist can also keep one hand on the patient's shoulder, ensuring the humeral head is rotated inwardly and the arm is either on the film holder or down behind the film holder.
  - The technologist uses her other hand to lift the breast up and out as compression is applied with the foot pedal.
  - The hand on the humeral head can also be used to pull the upper skin (just inferior to the clavicle), minimizing skin fold development.
- Pectoral muscle should be seen to the level of the nipple.
- If the pectoral muscle is relaxed appropriately, mobilized medially, and maintained medially during exposure, the pectoral muscle edge will have a convex contour.

- If the pectoral muscle edge is concave, parallel to the edge of the film, or triangular, the breast is not positioned optimally. The right angle of obliquity was not selected; the muscle was not relaxed adequately, mobilized medially, or, if mobilized, not maintained medially mobilized; or the patient backed out of the unit slightly.

- The pectoralis minor muscle is seen in a few women as a triangular density superimposed on the uppermost portion of the pectoralis major muscle.

- In women with Poland's syndrome, pectoral muscle is not seen on the MLO view and breast size may be asymmetric (small breast on the affected side).

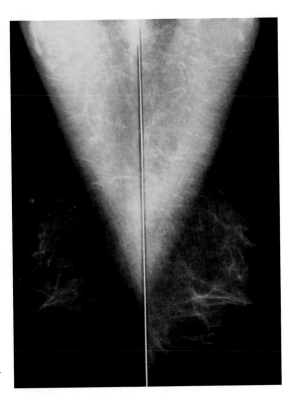

FIGURE 3-8
Right and left mediolateral oblique views corresponding to the craniocaudal views on Figure 3-4. Convex pectoral muscles extending to level of nipple.

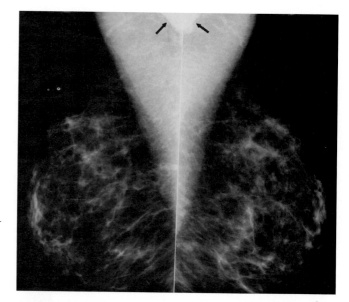

FIGURE 3-9
Right and left mediolateral oblique views corresponding to the craniocaudal views on Figure 3-5. Convex pectoral muscles extending to level of nipple. Pectoralis minor muscles (*arrows*) are seen as small triangular densities superimposed on the pectoralis major muscle.

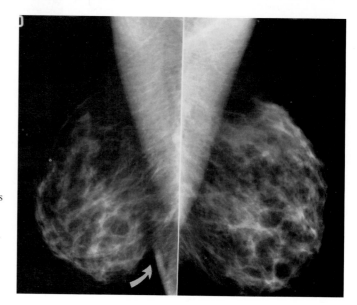

FIGURE 3-10
Right and left mediolateral oblique (MLO) views corresponding to the craniocaudal views on Figure 3-6. Convex pectoral muscles extending to level of nipple. Inclusion of too much abdomen on the right and failure to lift the breast up and out results in skin fold inferiorly (*arrow*). Including too much abdomen on MLO views can lead to blurring of tissue just above the inframammary fold (probably related to inadequate compression).

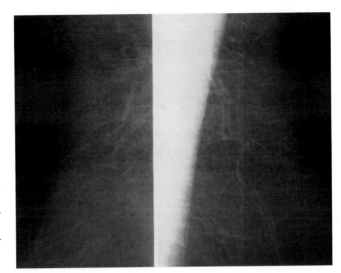

FIGURE 3-11
Poland's syndrome. Absence of pectoral muscle on the right. As in this patient, the breast on the affected side is usually smaller than the contralateral breast. Other ipsilateral chest wall abnormalities are sometimes identified in these patients, including supernumerary digits and absence of the nipple and clavicle.

Exaggerated Craniocaudal

KEY FACTS

- In approximately 10% of women, exaggerated CC views (uni- or bilateral) are done as part of the screening study to evaluate lateral tissue (prominent axillary tail of Spence).

- Indications
    - As part of the screening study: on CC views, tissue extends to the edge of the film laterally; on MLO views, a prominent tail of Spence is confirmed by seeing tissue extending superiorly, superimposed on pectoral muscle
    - To evaluate lateral lesions; may be combined with spot compression paddle

- This view is not accomplished by placing the film holder laterally, but rather by asking the patient to rotate so that the film holder can be placed at the mid-axillary line.

- For most women, the x-ray tube must be angled slightly so that the compression paddle does not come down on the humeral head. The tube must not be angled more than what is needed to clear the humeral head (5° maximum). If the tube is angled more, a shallow oblique view is obtained rather than a CC view.

- A small amount of pectoral muscle should be seen in all properly positioned exaggerated CC views.

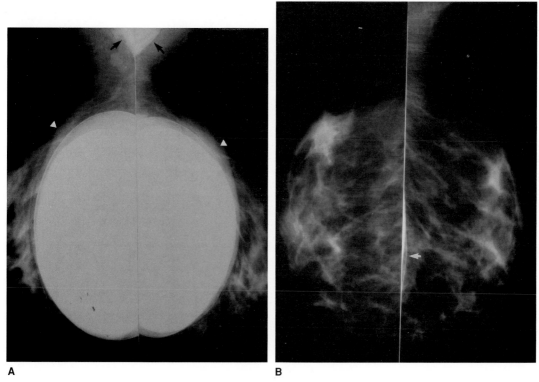

A   B

FIGURE 3-15   (**A**) Right and left mediolateral oblique (MLO) views. Subpectoral, double-lumen implant in the field of view. Pectoral muscle over implants (*arrowheads*). Pectoral minor muscles (*arrows*). (**B**) Right and left MLO implant-displaced views. Compressed tissue can now be evaluated. A small
amount of implant can be seen on the left (*arrow*).

(continued)

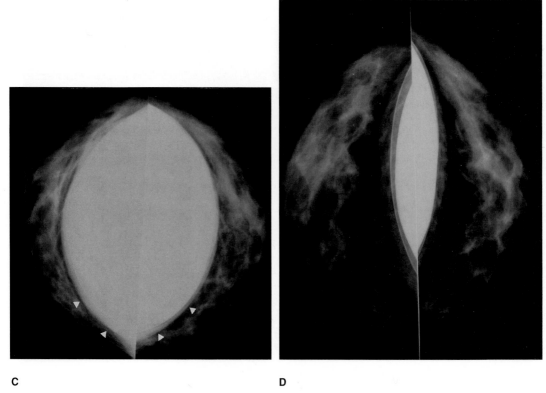

C   D

FIGURE 3-15   (**CONTINUED**) (**C**) Right and left craniocaudal (CC) views. Subpectoral, double-lumen implant in the field of view. Pectoral muscle overlying implants (*arrowheads*). (**D**) Right and left CC implant-displaced views.

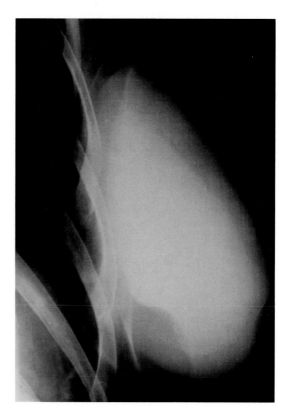

FIGURE 3-16
Chest wall view. The posterior aspect of implants is not seen with routine or implant-displaced views (see Fig. 3-15). The chest wall view can be done to evaluate the posterior portion of implants. This is done using an aluminum filter, no compression, and 38 to 42 kV.

Breast Compression and Anterior Compression Views

KEY FACTS

- Ideally, the breast is compressed until taut.

- Some women experience significant discomfort during compression. Compression should not be forced on patients: it is better to have suboptimal compression than an angry patient who leaves after an unpleasant experience and never returns to your facility or never has a mammogram at any facility again.

- The technologist should work with the patient by explaining the importance of compression and educating the patient on how long it will last. Let the patient know she is in control of the examination and of how much compression is applied: compression will be stopped when the breast is taut or at any point before that if the patient says so.

- Even when the patient tolerates compression, the base of the breast (the thickest part of the breast), the pectoral muscle, or the abdomen may limit compression of the anterior portion of the breasts. Whenever there is suboptimal compression, blur may degrade the images.

- Blur related to suboptimal compression can be focal. Evaluate the subareolar area, the edge of the pectoral muscles, and the trabecular pattern just above the inframammary fold. Do the structures look sharp? If there are calcifications or vessels, do they look sharp? If you suspect blur (motion), get additional views. You may want to use the spot compression paddle in the area of perceived blur.

- When anterior compression is compromised by a particularly thick breast base, prominent pectoral muscles, or too much abdomen in the field of view on the MLO view, or if anterior tissues are exposed inadequately, obtain anterior compression views.

- Anterior compression views are obtained by moving the compression paddle forward away from the base of the breast or the pectoral muscle. A spot compression paddle may be used if the area to be evaluated is small.

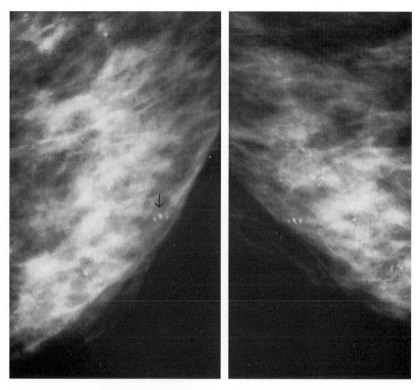

FIGURE 3-17   Blur. Right mediolateral oblique (MLO) views back to back photographi-
cally coned to the area just above the inframammary fold. There is blurring of the trabecular pattern (apparent loss of contrast; the tissue looks
whiter), and calcifications (*arrow*) localized to the area just above the inframammary fold (left image). Repeat MLO with attention to the inferior
portion of the beast improves resolution. More calcifications are now apparent and the trabecular pattern is sharper. If too much abdomen is included on MLO views, blurring just above the inframammary fold sometimes occurs.

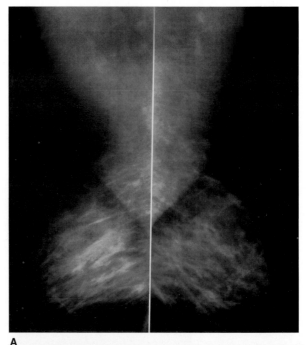

A

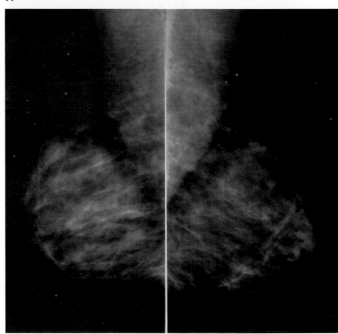

B

FIGURE 3-18

(**A**) Right and left mediolateral oblique (MLO) views. Strikingly prominent pectoral muscles. The anterior tissue is undercompressed. Underexposure of tissue on the right. (**B**) Anterior compression, right and left MLO views. Moving forward off the pectoral muscles so that compression of anterior tissue is optimized. In this patient, pectoral muscle is still seen (pectoral muscle is not always seen with anterior compression views). Although illustrated here with MLO views, this can also occur on craniocaudal views.

Spot Compression

KEY FACTS

- Indications
    - To establish or confirm the presence of a lesion: is this a lesion or is it normal superimposed tissue?
    - To evaluate masses more accurately (superimposed tissue obscuring the mass may be displaced)
    - To evaluate the subareolar area, particularly if the anterior portion of the breast is undercompressed
    - To obtain better exposure of a particularly dense area of tissue
- Focal compression is applied. The smaller paddle generally permits a greater degree of compression, helps spread tissue out, and brings the area of radiographic concern closer to the film, improving resolution.
- Assessing image quality
    - Well-exposed, high-contrast image
    - Include the area of concern on screening studies in the field of view. Sometimes lesions are compressed or squeezed out from under the spot compression paddle.
    - No motion, blurring

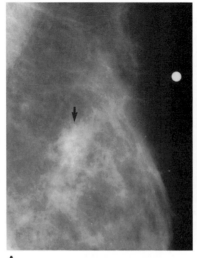
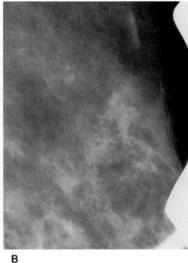

FIGURE 3-19
Superimposition. (**A**) Screening view with irregular density on mediolateral oblique (MLO) view superiorly. BB is marking skin lesion. (**B**) With spot compression, a lesion is effectively excluded. Superimposed glandular tissue accounts for density seen on the MLO view. When reviewing spot compression views, ascertain that the area of concern has not be pushed out of the field of view with compression.

A

B

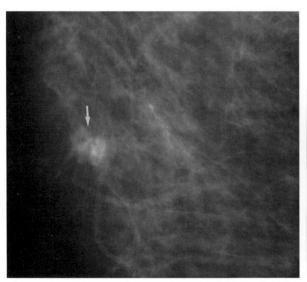
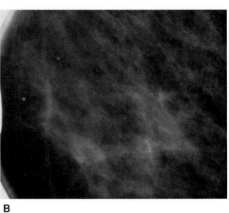

A

B

FIGURE 3-20   Superimposition. (**A**) Screening view with irregular density (*arrow*) on craniocaudal (CC) view medially. (**B**) With spot compression, a lesion is effectively excluded. Superimposed glandular tissue accounts for density seen on the CC view.

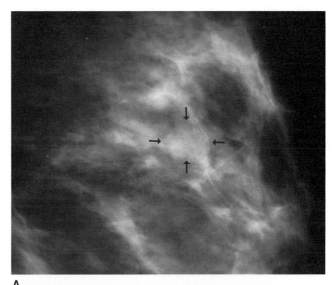

A

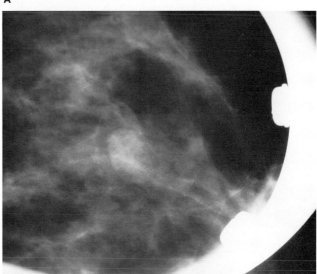

B

FIGURE 3-21

Fibroadenoma. (**A**) Possible mass detected on left craniocaudal screening view. Rounded contour is seemingly obscured by glandular tissue (*arrows*). (**B**) A well-circumscribed mass is confirmed after spot compression views. Spot compression facilitates focal compression so that tissue is spread apart and the area of concern is brought closer to the film to maximize resolution. (**C**) Solid hypoechoic mass on ultrasound. Fibroadenoma diagnosed by needle biopsy. This is the type of lesion that can be safely followed: probably benign lesion on spot compression views and ultrasound (see Chaps. 1 and 5).

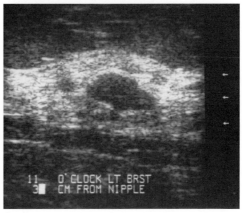

C

(Micro-Focal) Spot Magnification Views

KEY FACTS

- Indications
  - When there is a definite mass on the screening studies, magnification views may provide additional information on the margins, possible satellite lesions, and the presence or absence of associated microcalcifications.
  - When there are calcifications, magnification views provide more detailed morphologic information, additional calcifications in a given cluster may become apparent, and additional unsuspected clusters of calcifications may be detected.
  - Asymmetric tissue or areas of distortion may be further characterized.

- The full paddle or the spot compression paddle can be used. We prefer to use the spot compression paddle to maximize compression over the area of radiographic concern.

- For magnification, an air gap technique is used. As the breast is moved away from the film holder, magnification is obtained; increased distance from film means greater magnification. Magnification platforms of different heights are available; the maximal magnification is approximately 1.8 ×. To counter the effect of increased blurring at the edges related to the penumbra effect, a small focal spot (0.1 mm) is needed.

- No grid is used. Scatter radiation is dissipated in the air gap and therefore cannot degrade the image.

- Carbon-top magnification stands absorb radiation; a Lexan (polymer) top can be used instead of carbon to decrease the amount of radiation absorbed by the magnification stand itself by almost 20%, potentially improving image quality (because exposure times may be shortened, there is less likelihood of patient motion).

- Assessing image quality
  - Well-exposed, high-contrast image
  - No motion (this is a recurring problem for magnification views because of the relatively longer exposure times)
  - Area of concern imaged in two projections

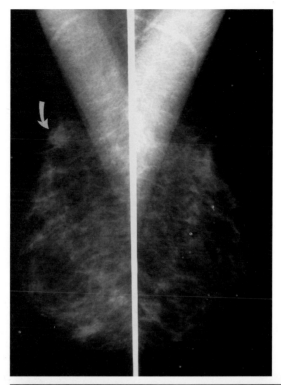

FIGURE 3-22
(**A**) Well-differentiated (low nuclear grade) ductal carcinoma in situ. Right and left mediolateral oblique (MLO) views. Minor low-density area of asymmetric tissue on the right (*arrow*). However, it is present in one of the critical areas of review. What would you say about this? Want more information? (**B**) Well-differentiated (low nuclear grade) ductal carcinoma in situ. Micro-focus (0.1 mm) spot magnification view (1.8 ×). Surprised? Ill-defined density with associated punctate microcalcifications. Even in retrospect, the calcifications cannot be seen on the routine MLO view. Well-differentiated (low nuclear grade) ductal carcinoma in situ with no associated invasion was found histologically. Recommendations can become much easier if thorough mammographic work-ups are undertaken.

B

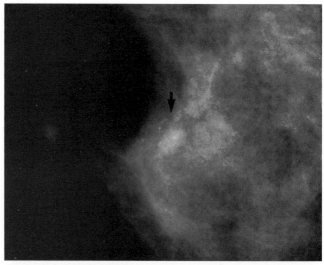

A

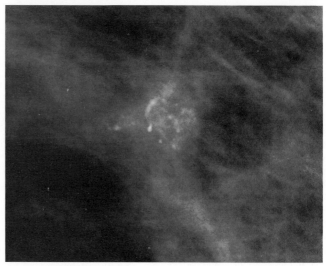

B

FIGURE 3-23

Intermediate- to high-grade ductal carcinoma in situ. (**A**) A few calcifications were identified on a screening study (*arrow*). Rather than attempting to characterize the calcifications on routine screening views, additional magnification views are recommended. (**B**) Microfocus (0.1 mm) spot magnification views (1.8 ×) confirm the presence of calcifications, demonstrate additional calcifications within cluster, and permit morphologic evaluation. Pleomorphic cluster of microcalcifications with punctate and linear calcifications requiring biopsy.

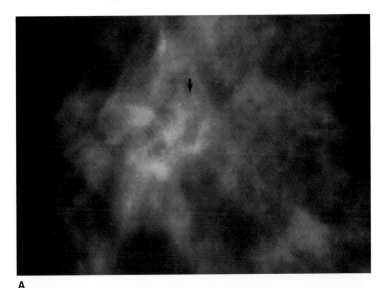

A

FIGURE 3-24
Mixed, well-differentiated and poorly differentiated ductal carcinoma in situ. (**A**) What appear to be calcifications were identified on a screening study. How much can we say about this finding and with what confidence? Rather than attempting to characterize the calcifications on routine screening views, additional (magnification) views are recommended. (**B**) Micro-focus (0.1 mm) spot magnification views (1.8 ×). More clusters and more calcifications within each imaged cluster are seen on the magnification views compared with the screening views. The clusters are composed of pleomorphic calcifications with predominance of punctate-type calcifications. High-yield biopsy recommendations are possible when lesions are appropriately evaluated.

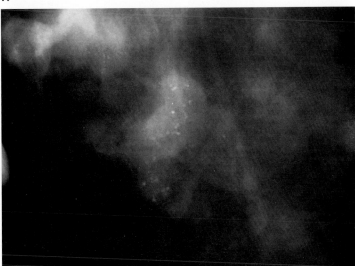

B

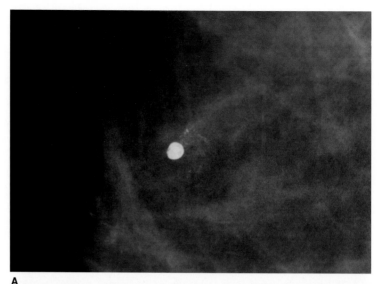

A

FIGURE 3-25
Well-differentiated and intermediately differentiated ductal carcinoma
in situ. (**A**) An area of calcifications
is seen on the screening view. Magnification views are recommended for
further characterization. (**B**) Micro-
focus (0.1 mm) spot magnification
views (1.8 ×). More calcifications
are identified within the cluster. Predominantly granular-type calcifications with pleomorphism. In the absence of linear form, this is unlikely
to be poorly differentiated ductal carcinoma in situ. The differential for
clusters like this includes well-differentiated ductal carcinoma in situ,
atypical ductal hyperplasia, sclerosing
adenosis, fibroadenoma, and papill-
loma.

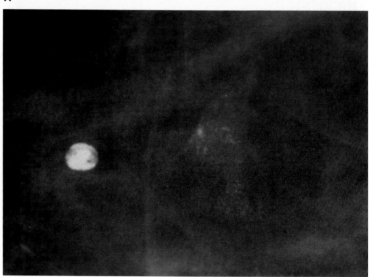

B

Tangential Views

KEY FACTS

- Indications
  - To demonstrate the dermal location of lesions (calcifications or masses)
  - In dense breast tissue, this view may improve detection and evaluation of palpable masses. Increased contrast can be obtained by surrounding the palpable area with subcutaneous, predominantly fatty tissue.
  - In post-lumpectomy and radiation therapy patients, this view can be used to separate skin changes from possible underlying post-lumpectomy changes (skin may project on lumpectomy site).
- A metallic BB is placed on the area of skin thought to contain calcifications or over the "lump" in symptomatic patients. This area is placed in a tangent to the x-ray beam. We use a spot compression paddle for these images.

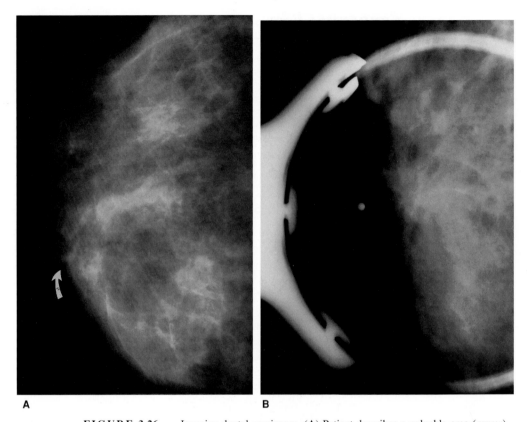

A   B

FIGURE 3-26   Invasive ductal carcinoma. (**A**) Patient describes a palpable area (*arrow*) medially on the right. Where is the metallic BB? Areas of clinical concern should be marked. We also routinely obtain tangential views of the area of clinical concern, particularly if there is tissue potentially obscuring the area. (**B**) Tangential view obtained. Metallic BB marks area of concern. A spiculated mass with architectural distortion becomes readily apparent. Rather than disclaim routine views and suggest "biopsy if clinically indicated" or "no obvious lesion mammographically; biopsy should be based on clinical findings," we can evaluate an area of clinical concern to completion, expediting the need for a biopsy in this patient.

Rolled Views (Change of Angle Views)

KEY FACTS

- As compared to normal breast tissue, which may change significantly in appearance as tissue is rolled, most breast cancers are three-dimensional. As tissue is rolled or the tube angle is changed, superimposed tissue may be rolled away, whereas breast cancers usually remain apparent.

- Rolled views can be done in any projection (eg, CC, MLO, 90° lateral), and tissue can be rolled in any direction desired. Depending on the surrounding tissue, the technologist may want to consider taking the area of the potential lesion and rolling it away from adjacent tissue (which may obscure the lesion) into a fatty area of the breast. This may make the lesion more conspicuous.

- As a rule, several rolled views are obtained, rolling the tissue in different direction and projections. Great care must be taken and the views reviewed thoroughly before saying there is no lesion.

- Rolled views are usually done with a spot compression paddle. However, any "extra" view of the breast represents a change of angle or a rolled view, because unless extra views are done without releasing compression, it is hard to reproduce breast positioning on any two views.

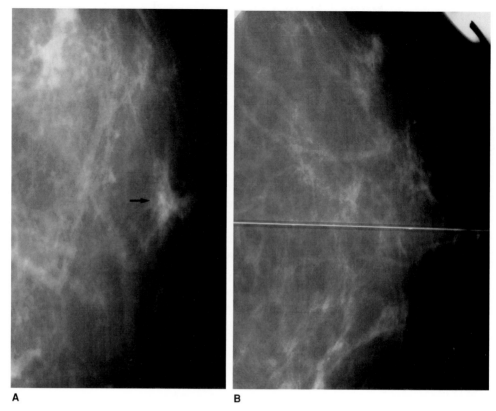

A   **B**

FIGURE 3-27   (**A**) Rolled views. Asymmetric tissue (*arrow*) on routine screening view. (**B**) Two rolled spot compression views back to back. Asymmetric tissue is spread out and changes configuration between views.

FIGURE 3-28
Spot compression and rolled spot compression views back to back. Asymmetric tissue (*arrow*) in upper portion of breast changes significantly between views. No underlying mass or architectural distortion is evident.

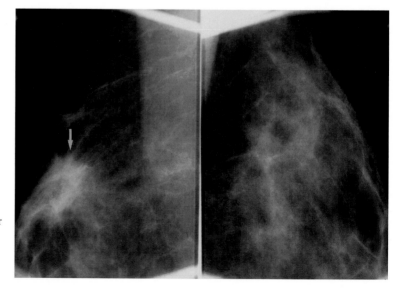

90° Mediolateral View

KEY FACTS

- A true 90° lateral view of the breast—because tissue is not being pulled away from the body parallel to the underlying muscle fibers, some tissue is probably excluded from the field of view

- The direction of the x-ray beam is defined by the name of the view. In this case, the x-ray beam enters the medial portion of the breast, traverses the breast, and exits on the lateral side onto the film.

- This is not a routine screening view, but rather a trouble-shooting view.

- Indications
  - Lateral lesion evaluation: the lateral portion of the breast is closest to the film, maximizing resolution
  - For preoperative needle localization and, in conjunction with the CC view, for determining the shortest distance from the skin to the lesion
  - In the triangulation of lesions seen on the CC view but not identified with certainty on the MLO view (or seen on the MLO view but not identified with certainty on the CC view)

90° Lateromedial View

KEY FACTS

- A true 90° lateral view of the breast—because tissue is not being pulled away from the body parallel to the underlying muscle fibers, some tissue is probably excluded from the field of view

- In this case, the x-ray beam enters the breast on the lateral side (compression paddle on the lateral portion of the breast) and exits the medial side (bucky and film on medial side) onto the film.

- This is not a routine screening view, but rather a trouble-shooting view.

- Indications

    - Medial lesion evaluation: the medial portion of the breast is closest to the film, maximizing resolution

    - If there is any question of medial tissue exclusion on the MLO view, the film holder is placed against the sternum (the patient is asked to extend her neck and rest her chin on top of the bucky), maximizing visualization of the medial portion of the breast

    - For preoperative needle localization and, in conjunction with the CC view, for determining the shortest skin-to-lesion distance

    - In the triangulation of lesions seen on the CC view but not identified with certainty on the MLO view (or seen on the MLO view but not identified with certainty on the CC view)

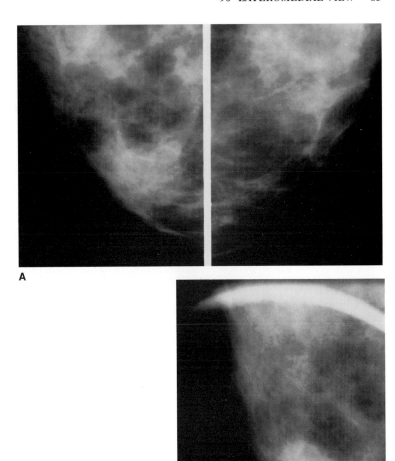

FIGURE 3-29
(**A**) Right and left craniocaudal (CC) views. Asymmetric tissue on the right medially. As in this patient, medial tissue on CC views should be examined and attention given to any developing density or asymmetry. (**B**) Spot compression CC projection confirms the presence of an ill-defined irregular mass medially on the right.

(continued)

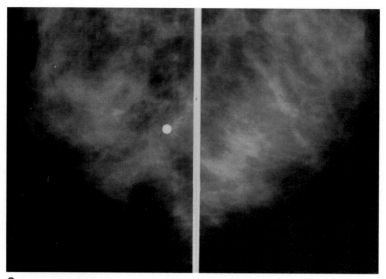

C
FIGURE 3-29
(CONTINUED)

(C) Right and left mediolateral oblique (MLO) views. Can you see the lesion with certainty on the right MLO? Has the mass been included in the field of view? What might you want to do next?

Lateromedial Oblique (True Reverse Oblique)

KEY FACTS

- Indications
    - Evaluation of medial lesions (medial tissue closest to film)
    - Patients with kyphosis, pectus excavatum, pectus carinatum, prominent pacemaker
    - Patients who recently underwent median sternotomy
- Beam travels from inferolateral to superomedial.
- Patient-specific angle is established as in routine MLO. The bucky is then placed just inferior to the clavicle and humeral head.
- Pectoral muscle should be relaxed.

Triangulation

KEY FACTS

- When a lesion is seen in only one view, every effort should be made to determine its location in another projection.

- By looking at the relative movement of a lesion between MLO (the screening view—the starting point) and 90° lateral views, the technologist can get a general idea of where the lesion is on the CC view.

  - If a lesion moves up in location from the MLO to the 90° lateral view, the lesion is in the medial half of the breast.

  - If a lesion moves down in location from the MLO to the 90° lateral view, the lesion is in the lateral half of the breast.

  - If a lesion does not shift much in position from the MLO to the 90° lateral view, the lesion is in the midportion of the breast behind the nipple.

- These same concepts can be applied if a lesion is identified in the CC view and its location is unclear in the MLO view.

  - A lateral lesion on the CC view moves down from MLO to 90° lateral view.

  - A medial lesion on the CC view moves up from MLO to 90° lateral view.

  - A lesion in the midportion of the breast does not shift between MLO and 90° lateral views.

  - See Figures 3-29 and 3-30.

BIBLIOGRAPHY

American College of Radiology. 1994. ACR standard for diagnostic mammography and problem solving breast evaluation. Reston, VA: author.

American College of Radiology. 1995. ACR standard for screening mammography. Reston, VA: author.

Bassett LW. Quality determinants of mammography: clinical image evaluation. RSNA Categorical Course in Breast Imaging Syllabus 1995; pp 57–67

Bassett LW, Hirbawi IA, DeBruhl N, Hayes MK. Mammographic positioning: evaluation from the view box. Radiology 1993;188:803–806

Bradley FM, Hoover HC, Hulka CA, et al. The sternalis muscle: an unusual normal finding seen on mammography. AJR 1996;166:33–36

Eklund GW, Busby RC, Miller SH, Job JS. Improved imaging of the augmented breast. AJR 1988;151:469–473

Eklund GW, Cardenosa G. The art of mammographic positioning. Radiol Clin North Am 1992;30:21–53

Eklund GW, Cardenosa G, Parsons W. Assessing adequacy of mammographic image quality. Radiology 1994;190:297–307

Meyer JE, Stomper PC, Lee RR. Pectoralis muscles simulating a breast mass. AJR 1989; 152:481–482

Samuels TH, Haider MA, Kirkbride P. Poland's syndrome: a mammographic presentation. AJR 1996;166:347–348

Sickles EA. Practical solutions to common mammographic problems: tailoring the examination. AJR 1988;151:31–39

Swann CA, Kopans DB, McCarthy KA. Localization of occult breast lesions: practical solutions to problems of triangulation. Radiology 1987;163:557

Breast Imaging Companion
by Gilda Cardenosa
Lippincott-Raven Publishers, Philadelphia © 1997

Chapter 4

TECHNICAL CONSIDERATIONS

General Comments

KEY FACTS

- High-quality mammographic images are critical if we expect to detect early cancers reliably.
- High quality requires an ongoing evaluation of images on a film-by-film basis.
- Assess images
  - Positioning
  - Exposure of glandular tissue
  - Contrast
  - Blurring
  - Film labeling

Equipment

KEY FACTS

- X-ray spectrum
  - Bremsstrahlung
  - Characteristic emission
  - Target materials
  - Filtration

- Target materials
  - Molybdenum: 17.4 and 19.6 keV
  - Rhodium: 20.2 and 22.7 keV
  - Tungsten

- Filtration
  - Molybdenum filtration (0.03 mm): 20.0 keV K-edge
  - Rhodium: 23.2 keV K-edge
  - Yttrium

- Window
  - Beryllium does not absorb soft characteristic radiation.

- Heel effect
  - X-ray beam intensity on anode side less than on cathode side
  - Cathode side directed at base of breast (thicker portion of breast requires higher intensity)

- Focal spot
  - Actual focal spot: area on anode struck by electrons
  - Effective focal spot: x-ray beam projected toward patient and film
  - Routine: 0.3 mm or smaller
  - Magnification: 0.15 mm or smaller

- Source-to-image distance
  - Smallest focal spot with largest source-to-image distance while maintaining low exposures
  - 50 to 80 cm
  - Average: 60 to 65 cm

- Object-to-film distance
  - As small as possible
  - As the breast is raised away from the film, magnification is obtained and there is loss of resolution (penumbra effect).

(text continues on the next page)

Equipment *(Continued)*

- Generator
  - Single-phase: low-intensity radiation, increased exposure times (patient motion)
  - Three-phase: increased tube capacity (mA output), decreased exposure time
  - High frequency
  - Constant potential

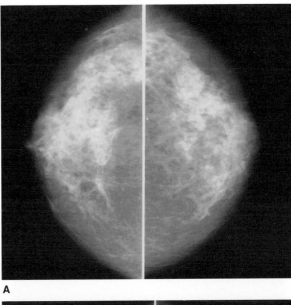

A

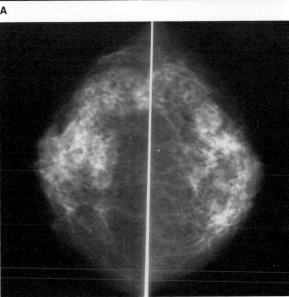

FIGURE 4-3
(**A**) Right and left craniocaudal (CC) views. Low
contrast. Gray images with visualization of subcutaneous tissue. (**B**) Right and left CC views. High-contrast images are optimal. Contrast is a function of
film type, processing (extended developing time for
some types of films), kV, optical density settings,
scattered radiation, and subject contrast.

B

Automatic Exposure Control (AEC)

KEY FACTS

- AECs control length of exposure required for desired image density.

- With kVp selected, adjustments in mAs compensate for breast thickness and tissue-type differences. Manual adjustment of exposure density is accomplished with the density knob.

- AEC must be able to determine if back-up time will be exceeded and should terminate exposure within 50 msec, 5 mAs, or at an entrance exposure (to ACR accreditation phantom) of less than 50 mR.

- AEC is adjusted for film/screen combination, processing, and cassettes in use.

- Position of AEC can be changed. Exposure reflects AEC positioning. If placed close to chest wall (retroglandular fat), anterior dense tissue may be underexposed; if positioned anteriorly, retroglandular fat may be overexposed.

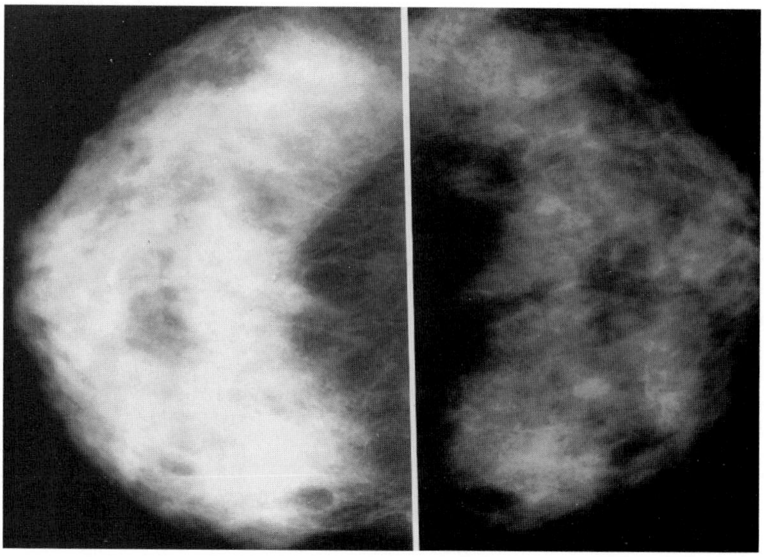

FIGURE 4-4
Right craniocaudal (CC) view with photo cell positioned posteriorly (close to chest wall) back to back with right CC view obtained with photo cell positioned anteriorly. The first image demonstrate adequate exposure of retroglandular fat, but anterior tissue is underexposed (unacceptably so). On the second image, retroglandular fat is overexposed but the glandular tissue is now adequately exposed (glandular tissue is being phototimed).

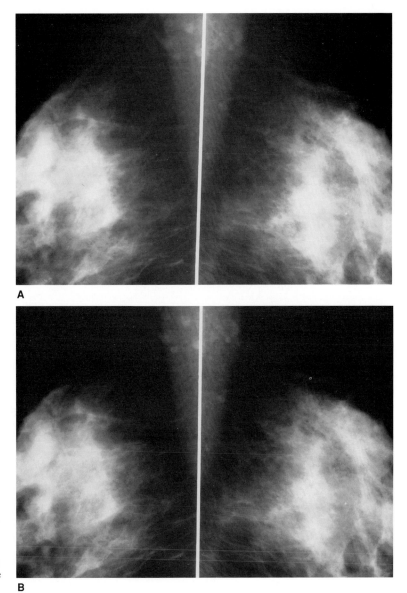

FIGURE 4-5
(**A**) Right and left mediolateral (MLO) views, photo cell close to chest wall. Retroglandular fat is adequately exposed, glandular tissue underexposed. (**B**) Right and left MLO views, middle photo cell position. Retroglandular fat is now overexposed, glandular tissue adequately exposed.

Grids

KEY FACTS

- Scatter radiation is detrimental to image quality and results in significant loss of contrast.
    - If no grid is used, scatter radiation can constitute 40% to 85% of primary beam intensity.
- Grids are used to absorb scatter radiation.
- Depending on the grid ratio, exposure times must be increased approximately 2.5 ×.
- Reciprocating grid (now industry standard)
    - 18 × 24 cm
    - 24 × 30 cm
    - Grid ratio: 3.5:1 to 5:1; usually 5:1 (32 lines/cm)

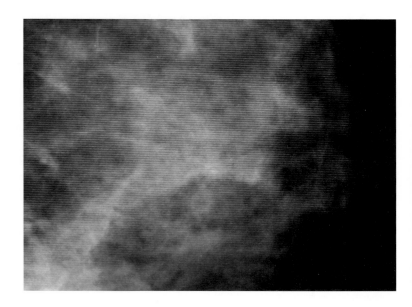

FIGURE 4-6
Grid lines.

Film

KEY FACTS

- Single-emulsion film
  - Film base: transparent plastic
  - Gelatin layers on both sides of film base
  - Emulsion (containing light-sensitive silver halide crystals; magenta dye—sensitizing film to green light; and chemicals for stability, low fog, and fast processing) on one side of film base only
  - Antiabrasive layer over emulsion to protect emulsion
  - On back, antihalation layer helps to prevent scatter and film curling during processing.
- Emulsion should be in contact with screen.
  - Manufacturers have notched film so that the technologist can place film in cassette correctly by feeling for the notches.
  - After loading the cassette with film, 15 minutes should be allowed to elapse, allowing for film settling and good contact before taking film of patient.
- Film characteristics described by H&D curve
  - High-contrast film is preferred for mammography (steepest curve).
  - Curve depends on processing environment.
  - Curve is independent of x-ray quality (kV, mA).
  - Curve is used to compare different film types or same film with different processing environments and to monitor daily processing conditions.

Processing

KEY FACTS

- Film processing is often the weakest link in producing high-quality mammographic images. It requires ongoing attention.
- Reciprocity law: film speed varies with exposure time
- Developer—latent image is developed
  - Developer temperature is specified by manufacturer (often 95°F) and should remain constant.
  - Time in developer: in 90-second processing, 19 to 23 seconds; can be extended to 45 seconds to improve development of latent image (extended developing processing time); need to work with film type and manufacturer
  - Chemical activity of solutions (specific gravity)
  - Agitation
- Fixer—image is fixed and unexposed and undeveloped silver halide is removed from film
- Wash—removes chemicals
  - May use a water filter
  - Algicides (depending on water supply)
- Dryer
- Solutions must be replenished. Replenishment rates depend on number of films being passed through processor.
- Solutions must be replaced. See manufacturer's specifications.

Viewboxes and Viewing Conditions

KEY FACTS

- High-luminance viewboxes should be used for interpretation of mammographic images (luminance of 3500 NIT compared with 1500 NIT luminance for regular x-ray viewboxes)
- Bulbs should be changed routinely (every 18 to 24 months), as luminance declines with use.
- If one bulb needs to be replaced, all bulbs should be replaced at once.
- Viewboxes and magnifying lens should be kept clean.
- A mechanism is needed to mask off extraneous light. The only light in the reading room should be coming through the mammographic images. If this is impossible, consider purchasing or making a viewing cone to block extraneous light.
- No circular coning should be done on routine screening studies. Circular coning around the breast precludes effective masking of extraneous light. This type of coning accomplishes nothing and can be detrimental during interpretation.

Artifacts

KEY FACTS

- X-ray equipment
    - Filter (corrosion, damaged, wrong filter)
    - Compression paddle (lip of paddle)
    - Image receptor holder (textured, paint, motion)
    - Grid (uneven motion, grid hesitation, very short exposure time, grid not plugged in, edge of grid on chest wall)
- Patient
    - Deodorant
    - Hair, hair products
    - Jewelry
    - Tattoo
    - Body part projecting on images (earlobe, chin, gown, arm)
- Cassette, film, or screen
    - Film scratches, nail dents (crimp)
    - Finger pressure (fingerprints)
    - Moisture
    - Screen scratches
    - Film loaded in cassette upside down
    - Upside-down cassette (in bucky)
    - Fog
    - Static
    - Foreign object on screen (dust, lint, small objects) affects film/screen contact.

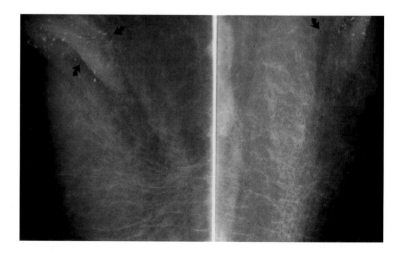

FIGURE 4-8
Deodorant. Right and left mediolateral oblique views. Deodorant can simulate malignant-type microcalcifications. Not usually a problem when seen in the axilla, but occasionally encountered at base of breast on craniocaudal views secondary to deodorant application in the inframammary fold area.

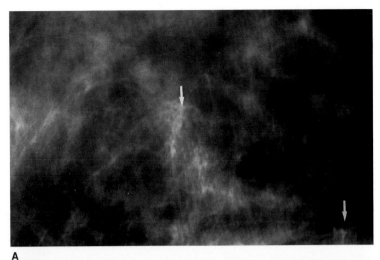

A

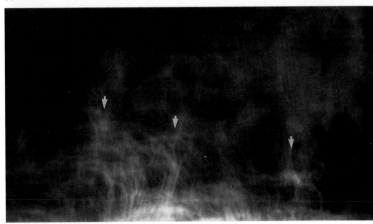

B

FIGURE 4-9
(A) Hair. Swirly appearance (*arrows*) common on craniocaudal (CC) views close to chest wall. (B) Hair, CC view. Swirly, blurry appearance close to chest wall.

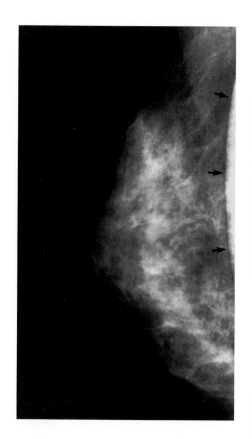

FIGURE 4-10
Right mediolateral oblique view. Skin fold
(*arrows*) projecting on pectoral muscle.

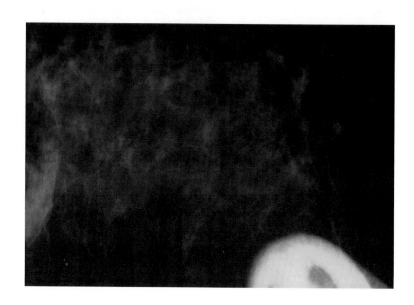

FIGURE 4-11
Nose artifact.

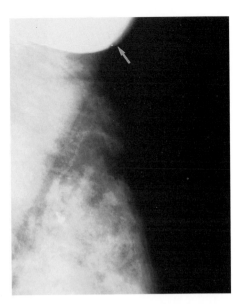

FIGURE 4-12
Chin (*arrow*). At this location you can sometimes see portions of the arm. If the arm interposes itself between the compression paddle and the bucky, compression may be limited and soft-tissue artifact is seen.

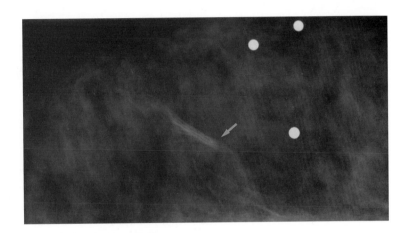

FIGURE 4-13
Garment artifact (*arrow*).

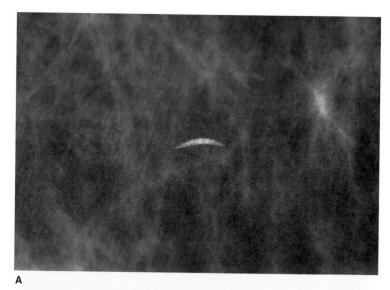

A

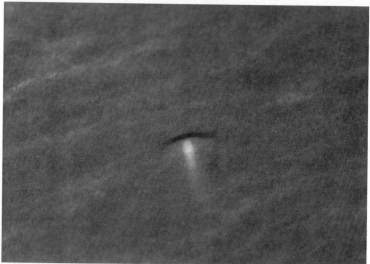

B

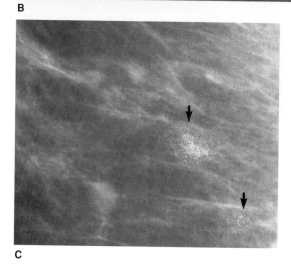

C

FIGURE 4-14
(**A**) Nail film crimp. Minus artifact
(before exposure). On inspection,
film is bent at this point. (**B**) Nail
film crimp. Plus artifact (after exposure). On inspection, film is bent at
this point. (**C**) Fingerprints (*arrows*).
Minus artifact (before exposure). Fingerprints can simulate microcalcifications.

(continued)

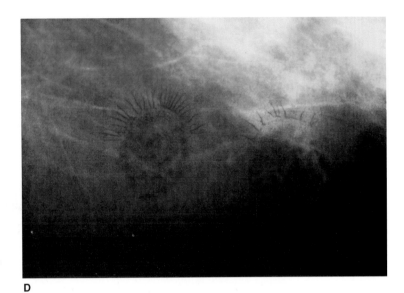

FIGURE 4-14
(CONTINUED) (D) Film handling (not quite fingerprints) with associated static ("ladybugs"). Plus artifact (after exposure).

D

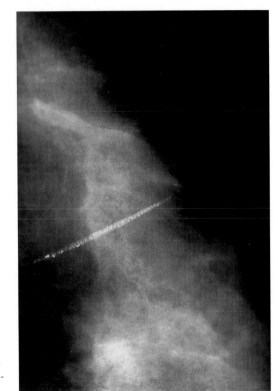

FIGURE 4-15
Nail polish. In our facility nail polish may not be worn by the technologists.

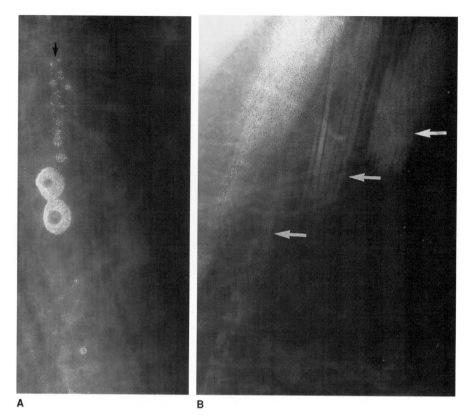

A

B

FIGURE 4-16   (**A,B**) Moisture (*arrows*). May be related to incomplete drying of cassette
after cleaning or to processor.

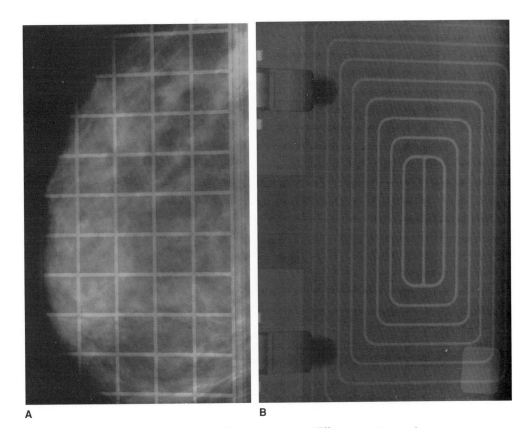

A   B

FIGURE 4-17   (**A,B**) Upside-down cassette (different cassette types).

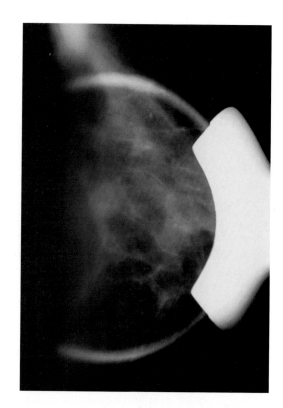

FIGURE 4-18
Poor film/screen contact (blurring) and fogged film, thought to be related to improper placement of film in cassette.

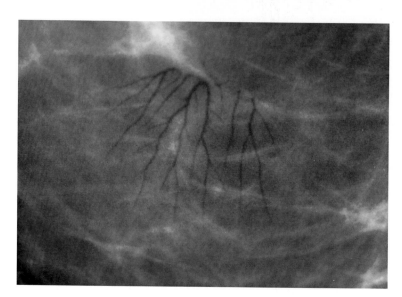

FIGURE 4-19
Static—focal fog (mammographic "lighting").

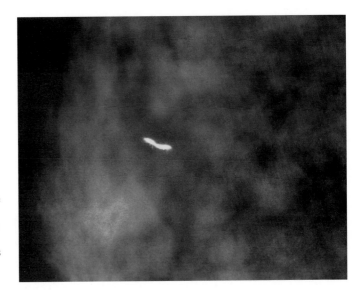

FIGURE 4-20
Poor film/screen contact. An object on the screen precludes close apposition between screen and film. The object can generally be seen (as in this case) as an artifact, and if the film is examined closely blurring can be seen surrounding the artifact. The blurring reflects poor film/screen contact. The film is actually lifted away from the screen by the artifact.

Processor Artifacts

KEY FACTS

- Processor: need to know
  - Plus or minus density artifact
  - Orientation of artifact (parallel, perpendicular, or random) with respect to direction of film travel
  - Emulsion orientation (emulsion side up or down)
  - Position of film on feed tray (right or left side of the processor)
  - Sensitometry
- Plus density (dark): developer stage; pressure or handling before exposure
- Minus density (light): fixer or wash; pressure or handling after exposure
- Processor: parallel to direction of film travel
  - Entrance roller marks: plus density, evenly spaced
  - Guide shoe marks: plus or minus density, evenly spaced, leading or trailing edge of film
  - Delay streaks: plus density, randomly spaced
- Processor: perpendicular to direction of film travel
  - Stub lines or hesitation lines: plus density, $1\frac{5}{8}''$ from leading edge
  - Chatter: plus density, evenly spaced
  - Slap lines: plus density, broad line $2\frac{1}{8}''$ to $2\frac{1}{4}''$ from trailing film edge
  - Pi lines
- Random artifacts
  - Drying patterns and water spots: seen with reflected light—mottled bands or spots
  - Wet pressure marks: plus density, resemble noise/quantum mottle
  - Runback: plus density, trailing edge of film
  - Flame pattern
  - Pickoff: minus density, small, emulsion removed down to film base

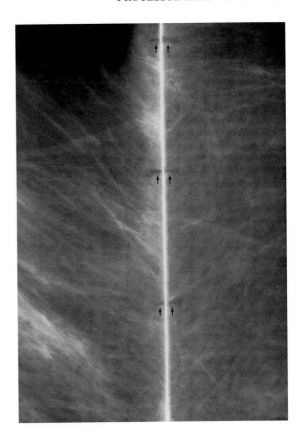

FIGURE 4-21
Guide shoe marks (*arrows*). Plus
density artifact, evenly spaced.

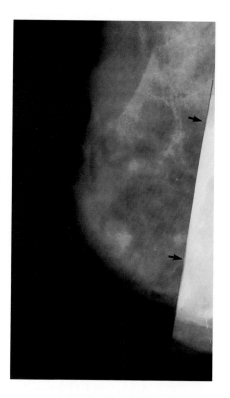

FIGURE 4-22
Overlap of films during processing, due to impatience. The first film is not completely into the processor before the second film is fed in (*arrows*).

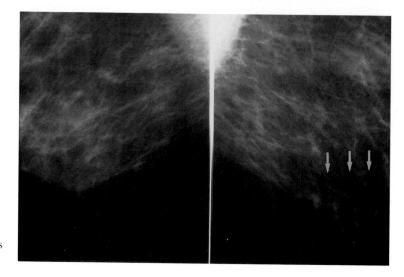

FIGURE 4-23
Fog. Evenly spaced. Darkroom light was turned on before film was completely in the processor.

BIBLIOGRAPHY

Bassett LW. Quality determinants of mammography: clinical image evaluation. RSNA Categorical Course in Breast Imaging Syllabus 1995; pp 57–67

Eklund GW, Cardenosa G, Parsons W. Assessing adequacy of mammographic image quality. Radiology 1994;190:297–307

Wentz G, Parson WC. Mammography for radiologic technologists. New York, McGraw-Hill, 1992

Widmer JH, Lillie RF, Jaskulski SM, Haus AG. Identifying and correcting processing artifacts. Technical and Scientific monograph #4, Eastman Kodak Company, 1994

Yaffe MJ, Hendrick RE, Feig SA, Rothenberg LN, Och J, Gagne R. Recommended specifications for new mammography equipment: report of the ACR-CDC focus group on mammography equipment. Radiology 1995;197:19–26

Ultrasound Artifacts

KEY FACTS

- Image distortion is related to variation in the speed of sound waves.
  - Ultrasound units assume the speed of sound is the same in different tissue types. However, the speed of sound is 1450 m/sec in fat and 1540 m/sec in soft tissue.
  - Therefore, traveling through fat takes longer than traveling through soft tissue. Increased transmission time means increased distance: the object appears deeper than it may actually be if different tissue types are crossed by the beam.
  - If the speed is greater than 1540 m/sec, the object may appear foreshortened.

- Phantom images related to refraction
  - These are generated because of the assumption that the ultrasound beam travels in a straight line.
  - If the beam is refracted and then hits a reflecting object, the echo retraces its oblique path back to the transducer. Because the assumption is that the beam is traveling in a straight line, the object is displayed at an appropriate distance directly down from the transducer.

- Blurring related to finite beam width
  - Blur depends on the width of the ultrasound beam at particular depths. Objects smaller than the ultrasound beam appear larger. The size seen depends on the beam width at the given lesion depth. The object is sharpest and most narrow (closest to its actual size) when the depth of the object is at the focal depth for the transducer (narrowest beam point).

- Distorted images of interfaces are related to finite beam width.
  - At an interface, two regions of a structure are at different depths. These echoes are treated as though arising from one position along the central axis of the beam.
  - The image depicts echo sites directly behind one another when in fact they are not. The interface is therefore distorted.

- "Fill-in," partial volume effect, is also related to finite beam width.
  - Echoes are detected from areas outside the central beam axis.
  - This is why small cysts contained entirely in the beam width may not be seen at all or may contain internal echoes. The acoustic properties of cysts differ from those of adjacent tissue, and partial volume effect occurs.

- Reverberation
  - This is due to impedance mismatch between the transducer and the patient's skin. Part of the beam is reflected back into the patient.

(text continues on the next page)

Ultrasound Artifacts (Continued)

- • There are two interfaces within the breast. Echoes from the two interfaces, displayed correctly, are followed by repeating artifactual echoes separated by equal distances (the distance between the interfaces), decreasing in amplitude.
- • These reverberation artifacts can result in ''filling in'' of cysts and mirror images.

- Posterior acoustic enhancement and shadowing, although useful in evaluating lesions, can also be considered artifactual.
  - • It is assumed that the same TGC curve is applicable to all scan lines generating an image.
  - • However, this is not necessarily true when scanning through a cyst (ie, nonattenuating compared with surrounding tissue) or when scanning through an infiltrating lobular carcinoma (lesions that can significantly attenuate the sound beam compared with surrounding tissue).

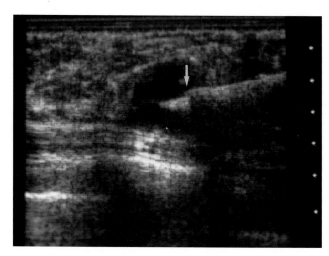

FIGURE 5-1
Bayonet sign. Given differences in the speed of sound between tissue and fluid in cyst, the needle appears broken (*arrow*). This confirms the presence of the needle within the fluid-filled structure. If not seen, the needle may still be in the cyst; if seen, however, one can be certain the needle is in the cyst.

Scanning

KEY FACTS

- Patient positioning
  - Breast tissue should be thinned maximally for adequate penetration with high-frequency transducer.
  - Most common starting position is supine contralateral posterior oblique. Depending on breast size and lesion location, however, the degree of obliquity can be changed as needed to thin tissue maximally.
  - The ipsilateral arm is elevated, helping to thin and spread tissue.
  - One of the advantages of ultrasound is that positioning can be changed as needed to evaluate a particular area or a given symptom in the breast.
  - Supine positioning may facilitate evaluation of the medial portion of the breast.
  - Upright positioning is needed if a lesion is palpable only when the patient is upright.
- Compression of tissue with transducer
  - To thin tissue
  - To assess compressibility of lesion—benign lesions are more compressible than malignant
  - To eliminate critical angle shadowing (which can preclude evaluation of deeper tissue) from superficial Cooper's ligaments
  - Too much compression may be counterproductive by causing patient discomfort, by pushing lesions out of the scan plane, or by altering the focal zones so that superficial lesions might be missed.
- TGC
  - Fatty tissues should be medium gray from skin to pectoral muscle.
  - Shallow curve for fatty tissue; steeper curve for glandular tissue
  - Depth should be enough to see pectoralis muscles, rib, and pleural line.
- Transducer manipulation
  - Transducer should be moved slowly with one hand as correlative physical examination is undertaken with the contralateral hand. The examiner's fingers can move back and forth at the leading edge of the transducer, correlating what is seen with what is felt.
  - If a potential lesion is identified, the transducer should be moved back and forth and rotated at least 90° to ensure that what is being seen is not a fatty lobule in cross section.
- Although breast ultrasound is targeted to the area of palpable or mammographic concern, a wider section of tissue surrounding the area of the lesion should be evaluated.

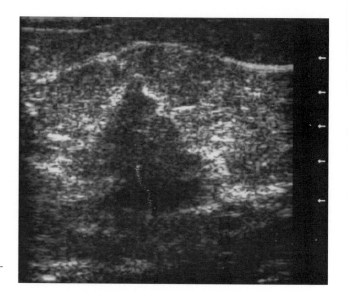

FIGURE 5-2
Critical angle shadowing associated with Cooper's ligaments. This may be confused with a lesion. The transducer angle must be changed or the radiologist must compress over the area to exclude a lesion.

Normal Anatomy

KEY FACTS

- Unlike fat elsewhere in the body, fat in the breast is hypoechoic relative to glandular tissue.
  - In mammographically dense tissue, ultrasound is helpful because hypoechoic lesions are readily discernible from adjacent relatively hyperechoic glandular tissue.
  - In mammographically fatty tissue, even lesions 1 to 2 cm may not be apparent on ultrasound because the echo pattern of the lesion may not be significantly different from that of the surrounding fat. In other words, the lesion is isoechoic with surrounding tissue.

- Skin
  - With the stand-off pad (so as to place the skin in the correct depth of focus for the transducer), a hypoechoic central area is sandwiched between two echogenic bands measuring approximately 13 mm wide.

- Ribs
  - Depending on how the transducer is held and the orientation of the underlying ribs, these may be seen as linear, hyperechoic bands with posterior acoustic shadowing or as oval, repeating hypoechoic masses. A novice may mistake the latter for a lesion. In fact, ribs can serve as good example for a patient who wants to see what a ''tumor'' looks like or how a tumor differs from a cyst.

- Pectoral muscles
  - Pectoralis major and minor muscles seen as one
  - Hypoechoic bands of variable widths with specular echoes overlying ribs
  - Thin hyperechoic band—the deep pectoral fascia overlying the pectoral muscles separates muscle from overlying breast tissue.

- Ligaments
  - Hyperechoic bands of variable thickness crisscrossing breast tissue
  - May generate areas of irregular shadowing; compression may eliminate this shadowing

- Lymph nodes
  - Well-circumscribed, hypoechoic mass with hyperechogenic focus (fatty hilum)

- Tissue
  - Bundles of fatty and glandular tissue interposed among fibrous bands (Cooper's ligaments)

(text continues on the next page)

Normal Anatomy (Continued)

- Depending on how the transducer is held, these tissue bundles can be seen longitudinally or as potential masses when viewed in cross section (as the transducer is rotated 90°). When a potential lesion is seen, rotate the transducer over it. If it is a "pseudolesion," it will take on a longitudinal appearance and fuse with surrounding tissue. If it is a true lesion, it will maintain its rounded or oval shape, remaining distinct from surrounding tissue.
- May see ductal structures when imaging close to the nipple
- If ducts are traced away from the nipple, they thin out and can sometimes be seen connecting to small hypoechoic masses (presumably acini).

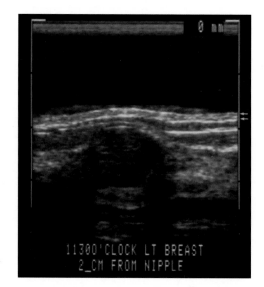

FIGURE 5-3
Normal skin; fibroadenoma. Skin is made up of a hypoechoic band sandwiched between two hyperechoic bands (*white arrows*). Hypoechoic mass (fibroadenoma).

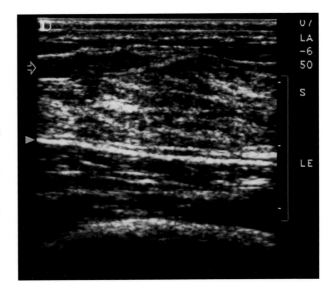

FIGURE 5-4

Rib (*arrow*), pectoral muscles, deep pectoral fascia (*arrowhead*), glandular tissue (fibrous tissue), and fat lobules (*open arrow*). Ribs in cross section are oval, repeating hypoechoic structures. The pectoral muscles are hypoechoic bands of variable width (depending on what part of the breast is being imaged), with linear or punctate high specular echoes separated from overlying breast tissue by a hyperechoic band (*arrowhead*), the deep pectoral fascia. Glandular tissue is hyperechoic, fatty tissue hypoechoic. Echogenicity, as described by Stavros, is relative to the echogenicity of subcutaneous fat.

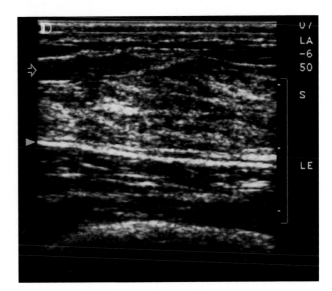

FIGURE 5-5

Deep pectoral fascia (*arrowhead*, hyperechoic band) separates the pectoral muscles from overlying glandular and fatty tissue. Echogenic glandular tissue, hypoechoic fatty tissue (fat lobule, *open arrow*). Ribs are not readily apparent on this image.

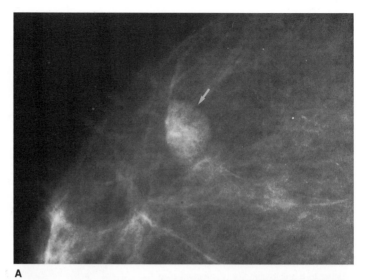

A

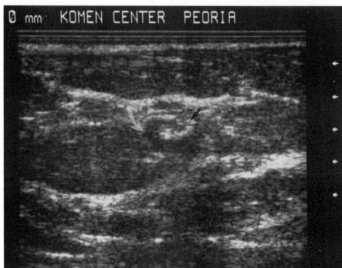

FIGURE 5-6
Lymph node. (**A**) Well-defined mass. Possible fatty hilum is seen mammographically (*arrow*). (**B**) Hypoechoic mass (*curved arrow*) with hyperechogenic area (*arrow*, fatty hilum) confirms this as a lymph node.

B

FIGURE 5-7
Diagram illustrating the importance of rotating the transducer during ultrasound evaluation of breast tissue. Bundles of breast tissue are intercalated within the skeleton provided by Cooper's ligaments. As the transducer is rotated 90°, a mass-like lesion may be seen (ie, the bundle in cross section). A true lesion remains discrete (oval, round, irregular) as the transducer is rotated.

BREAST ULTRASOUND

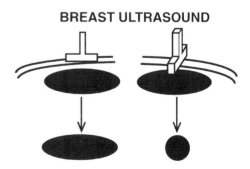

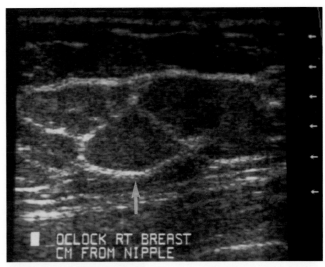

A

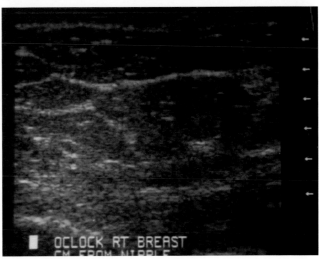

B

FIGURE 5-8
(**A**) ''Pseudolesion.'' In cross section, fatty tissue bundle is imaged as a round, mass-like area (*arrow*). Fixing on this area, the transducer should be slowly turned. If there is a true lesion, the shape will persist; if this is fatty lobulation, significant changes in its overall appearance can be expected. Ligaments are seen as hyperechoic bands. (**B**) As the transducer is rotated, the mass-like lesion is no longer seen. In real time, it can be seen fusing with surrounding tissue and becoming oblong.

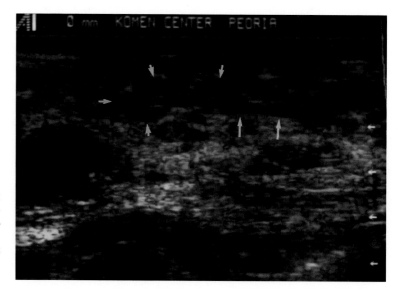

FIGURE 5-9

Duct (*long arrows*) can be followed back as it branches into small hypoechoic nodules (*small arrows*), probably acini. A cyst can be seen beyond and inferior to the lobular unit demonstrated. Cysts are fluid-filled, distended, and fused acini.

Benign Characteristics (Solid Masses)

KEY FACTS

- Hyperechogenicity
  - Tissue markedly hyperechoic relative to subcutaneous fat is fibrous tissue.
  - These fibrous ridges may be palpable.
  - Areas of fibrocystic change (fibrocystic complex) are hyperechoic with small (<0.5 cm) hypoechoic or anechoic nodules; these may also be palpable.

- Ellipsoid
  - Wider than tall; sagittal and transverse dimension greater than anteroposterior dimension

- Gentle bi- or trilobed

- Thin echogenic pseudocapsule
  - Slow-growing lesions
  - Real-time scanning (in different directions, moving the transducer back and forth along different planes) is usually needed to document complete "pseudo-capsule."

- Negative predictive value for sonographically benign classification of 99.5% reported by Stavros.
  - 1.6% of malignant lesions were misclassified as benign.
  - By excluding nodules with even one malignant-type finding, the reported sensitivity was 98.4%.

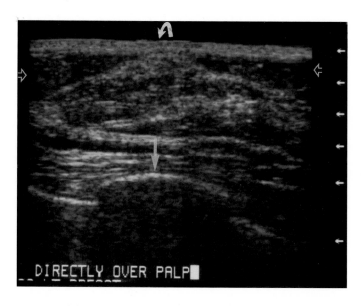

FIGURE 5-10
Palpable fibrous ridge. Fibrous tissue peak
(*curved arrow*) with fatty lobules (*open arrows*) on either side, described as a discrete mass by the patient and palpated by
the radiologist during the ultrasound examination. When areas such as this are seen
on ultrasound, correlating directly with the
area of palpable concern, biopsies can be
averted. Rib appears more linear than
mass-like (*large arrow*) in this scan.

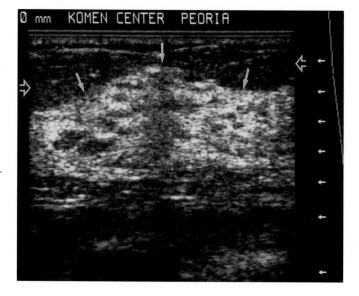

FIGURE 5-11
Palpable fibrocystic complex. Hyperechoic tissue (*arrows*) within which small round to
oval hypoechoic areas can be identified. Fibrous area peaks with fatty lobules (*open arrows*) on either side of peak. When scanning
the patient, this area is palpable as a distinct
lump. Biopsy in these patients can be averted
if this is all that is seen and it is correlated to
the palpable lump.

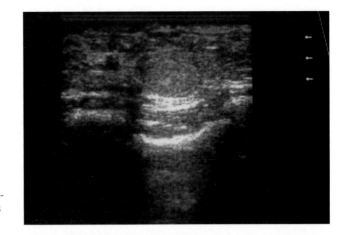

FIGURE 5-12
Hemorrhagic cyst. Hyperechoic mass with posterior acoustic enhancement. Hyperechogenicity is usually a benign finding.

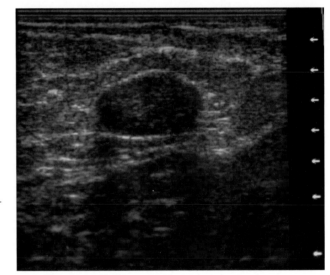

FIGURE 5-13
Fibroadenoma. Oval, hypoechoic mass with partial visualization of ''pseudocapsule'' (thin hyperechoic band around part of the lesion). During real-time scanning, as the transducer is rotated and gently manipulated from side to side, the pseudocapsule can be demonstrated surrounding the mass.

Intermediate Characteristics (Solid Masses)

KEY FACTS

- Isoechogenicity
  - Lesion seen mammographically or palpated not discernible as a cyst or solid mass
  - Can presume lesion is solid
- Mild hypoechogenicity
- Normal sound transmission
- Enhanced transmission
- Heterogeneous echotexture
- Homogeneous echotexture

Malignant Characteristics (Solid Masses)

KEY FACTS

- Marked hypoechogenicity

- Spiculation
  - Simulates spiculation seen mammographically
  - Alternating hyperechogenic and hypoechogenic bands radiating perpendicularly from mass
  - Thick echogenic halo seen around lateral edges also considered hypoechoic spiculation
  - Malignant characteristic with highest positive predictive value reported by Stavros

- Taller than wide
  - At least part of the nodule has a greater anteroposterior dimension than either sagittal or transverse.
  - Growth across normal tissue planes
  - Low sensitivity, high positive predictive value

- Angular margins
  - Junction between mass and surrounding tissue
  - Angle may be acute, obtuse, or right.
  - Reliable sign of malignancy

- Shadowing
  - Less through transmission of sound than surrounding tissue
  - Present even if mild or incomplete (associated with only part of the mass)

- Microlobulation
  - Many small (1 to 2 mm) lobulations on surface of mass

- Duct extension
  - Projection from mass radially in or around duct and coursing toward the nipple

- Calcifications
  - High specular echoes within mass

- Branch pattern
  - Multiple projections within or around ducts extending away from the nipple

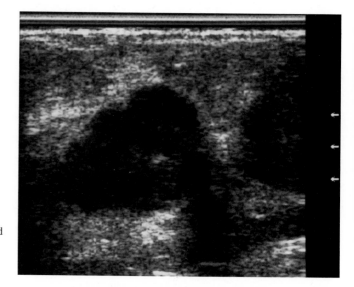

FIGURE 5-14

Infiltrating ductal carcinoma. Markedly hypo-echoic mass with lobulation, vertically oriented segments, and some shadowing. Malignant lesions usually exhibit several of the malignant characteristics described.

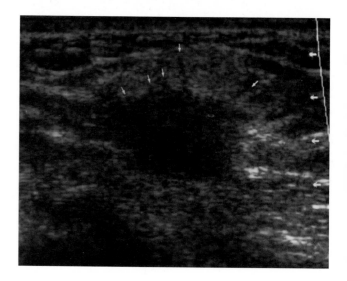

FIGURE 5-15

Infiltrating ductal carcinoma. Hypoechoic mass with spiculation (*arrows*).

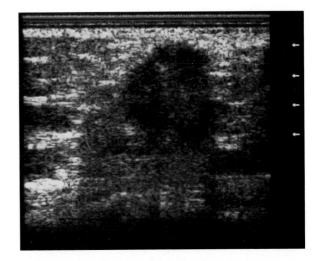

FIGURE 5-16
Infiltrating ductal carcinoma. Hypoechoic mass with posterior acoustic shadowing and vertical orientation.

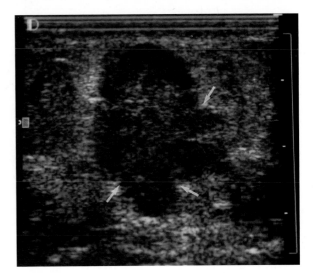

FIGURE 5-17
Infiltrating ductal carcinoma. Although heterogeneous, there are some areas of marked hypoechogenicity in this mass with angular (*arrows*) margins and vertical orientation.

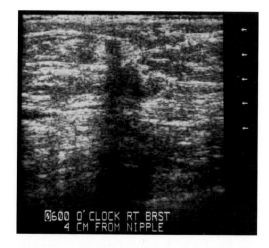

FIGURE 5-18
Infiltrating ductal carcinoma. Irregular hypoechoic mass with posterior acoustic shadowing.

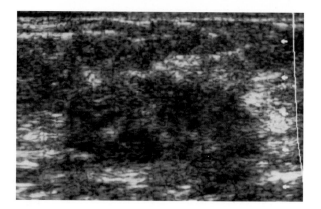

FIGURE 5-19
Infiltrating ductal carcinoma. Hypoechoic mass with lobulation.

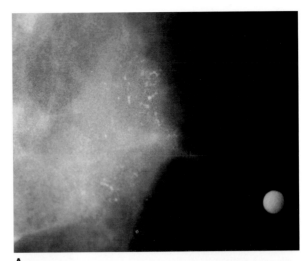

A

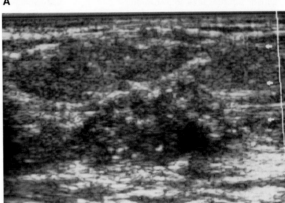

FIGURE 5-20
Infiltrating ductal carcinoma with associated high-grade ductal carcinoma in situ; (extensive intraductal component). (**A**) Pleomorphic cluster of linearly oriented and punctate microcalcifications. (**B**) Hypoechoic mass with high specular echoes (calcifications).

B

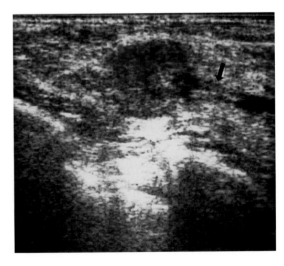

FIGURE 5-21
Infiltrating ductal carcinoma. Hypoechoic mass with posterior acoustic enhancement and extension into duct (*arrow*) toward nipple. Orientation to nipple established during real-time scanning.

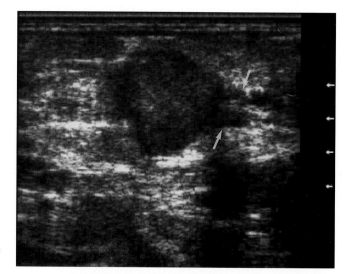

FIGURE 5-22
Infiltrating ductal carcinoma. Hypoechoic mass
with branch pattern—tubular pattern (*arrows*)
moving away from nipple. Orientation to nipple
established during real-time scanning.

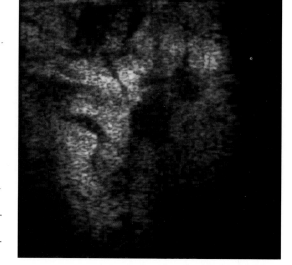

FIGURE 5-23
Inflammatory carcinoma, diffuse
breast involvement. Although no
discrete mass is identified, breast
anatomy and echo pattern are distorted completely, with irregular
areas of hyper- and hypoechogenicity throughout the breast associated with irregular tube-like structures.

BIBLIOGRAPHY

Bassett LW, Kimme-Smith C. Breast sonography. AJR 1991;156:449–455

Goodsitt MM, Ultrasound instrumentation and the A, B, M's of ultrasound. In Taveras JM, Ferrucci JT (eds). Radiology, diagnosis, imaging, intervention. Philadelphia, JB Lippincott, 1993

Gordon PB, Gilks B. Sonographic appearance of normal intramammary lymph nodes. J Ultrasound Med 1988;7:545–548

Jackson VP. The role of US in breast imaging. Radiology 1990;177:305–311

Jokich PM, Monticciolo DL, Adler YT. Breast ultrasonography. Radiol Clin North Am 1992; 30:993–1009

Kimme-Smith C, Rothchild PA, Bassett LW, Gold RH, Westbrook D. Ultrasound artifacts affecting the diagnosis of breast masses. Ultrasound Med Biol 1988;14(suppl):203–210

Stavros AT, Dennis MA. An introduction to breast ultrasound. In Parker SH, Jobe WE (eds). Percutaneous breast biopsy. New York, Raven Press, 1993, pp 95–109

Stavros AT, Dennis MA. The ultrasound of breast pathology. In Parker SH, Jobe WE (eds). Percutaneous breast biopsy. New York, Raven Press, 1993, pp 111–127

Stavros AT, Thickman D, Rapp CL, Dennis MA, Parker SH, Sisney GA. Solid breast nodules: use of sonography to distinguish benign and malignant lesions. Radiology 1995;196: 123–134

Venta LA, Dudiak CM, Salomon CG, Flisak ME. Sonographic evaluation of the breast. RadioGraphics 1994;14:29–50

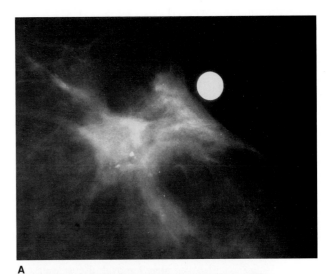

A

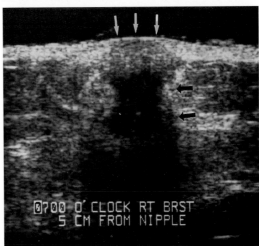

B

FIGURE 6-5
Infiltrating ductal carcinoma not otherwise specified. (**A**) Spiculated mass with skin thickening
and retraction. Microcalcifications reflect presence of associated ductal carcinoma in situ. Metallic BB placed in area of clinical findings. Inflammatory processes and postoperative changes
can produce similar findings. (**B**) Markedly hypoechoic mass (*black arrows*) with posterior acoustic shadowing. Disruption of the normal skin appearance (*white arrows*) and skin thickening
(offset pad used). (**C**) Spiculated mass extending
to skin. Subtle skin thickening directly under metallic BB (marking area of palpable mass) is appreciated on tangential view.

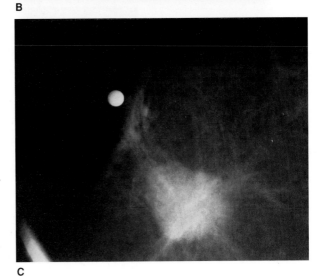

C

Epidermal and Sebaceous Cysts

KEY FACTS

- Clinical

  - Epidermal and sebaceous cysts are clinically indistinguishable.

  - Retention cysts: plugging of gland orifice with resultant keratin accumulation

  - Readily palpable, well-defined subcutaneous mass; can become large

  - May be visible, causing smooth skin bulge—orifice of the gland may be seen as a dark point

  - If squeezed, may see white, thick, cheesy material exuding from gland orifice

  - May become inflamed, particularly if ruptured

  - May need to be incised and drained. However, for epidermal cysts, adherence of cyst wall to surrounding tissue leads to recurrences (unless there is complete removal of cyst wall).

- Mammography

  - Well-defined mass. Because of its subcutaneous location, it may be apparent only under bright light. To get adequate exposure of glandular tissue, skin and subcutaneous tissues are usually "burned out."

  - Tangential view is helpful in demonstrating lesion and localizing to the skin.

  - May have associated calcifications

- Ultrasound

  - Superficial location (depending on transducer used, may need offset pad)

  - Attached to skin

  - May be completely anechoic, hypoechoic, or echogenic with posterior acoustic enhancement

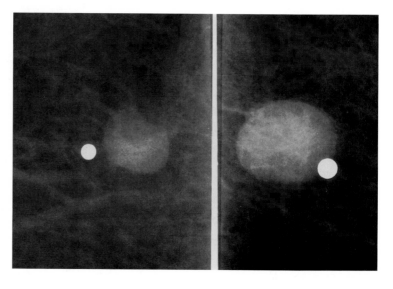

FIGURE 6-6
Sebaceous cyst. 1989 and 1993 left craniocaudal views, back to back. Well-defined mass projecting on breast parenchyma (metallic BBs indicate presence of subcutaneous palpable mass) As in this patient, sebaceous and epidermal cysts can change in size between examinations.

- Histology
  - Epidermal cysts: true epidermal cell lining with granular cell layer filled with keratin
  - Sebaceous cysts: epithelial cell lining, eosinophilic contents; may contain calcification

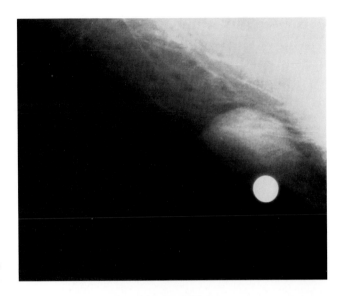

FIGURE 6-7
Sebaceous cyst. Well-defined mass seen in tangent to x-ray beam. Metallic BB used to indicate presence of subcutaneous, readily palpable mass.

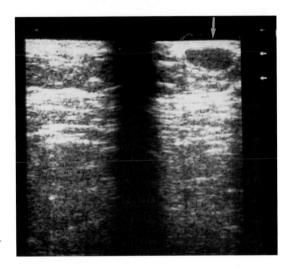

FIGURE 6-8
Sebaceous cyst. Hypoechoic, well-defined oval mass (*white arrow*) in subcutaneous tissue (offset pad used).

Neurofibromatosis

KEY FACTS

- Clinical
    - Autosomal dominant disease with high penetrance and variable expressivity; single gene (long arm chromosome 17) congenital syndrome affecting one in 2000 to 3000 persons
    - Heterogeneous disease with two distinct variants
    - Type I, von Recklinghausen's: most common phakomatosis—accounts for more than 90% of neurofibromatosis patients; cutaneous lesions more common in this type (but can also be seen in type II)
    - Café-au-lait, neurofibromas, neurilemomas
    - Neurofibromas involve neural plexus or peripheral nerve sheath.
    - Cutaneous lesions increase in size and number with advancing age.
    - Other possible diagnoses in patients with multiple skin lesions: Gardner's syndrome, cutaneous metastases, lipomatosis, steatocystoma multiplex, multiple leiomyomas, glomangiomas, xanthomatosis, cysticercosis

- Mammography
    - Multiple skin lesions—portion outlined by air is well defined
    - Evaluation of the breast may be difficult and limited because of skin lesions.

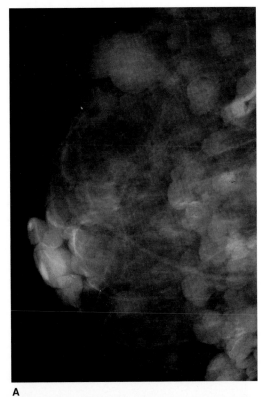

A

FIGURE 6-9
Neurofibromatosis. (**A**) Myriad skin lesions project on breast parenchyma. (**B**) Part of the lesions is well defined as outlined by air. The well-defined margin is lost where the lesions attach to the skin; black arrows denote transition point for margin definition for three skin lesions.

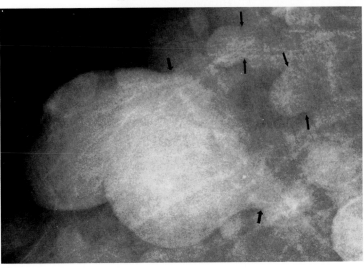

B

Mondor's Disease

KEY FACTS

- Clinical
  - Thrombophlebitis of a superficial vein of the breast (or the anterior chest wall). The thoracoepigastric vein is most commonly affected (traverses obliquely from epigastrium to anterior axillary line over lateral aspect of breast). The lateral thoracic vein, along the lateral margin of the pectoralis major, is involved less frequently.
  - Tender, cord-like structure associated with erythema and skin dimpling (particularly with arm elevation)
  - Limited benign condition; resolves spontaneously (2 to 24 weeks); no treatment necessary
  - Unknown cause: history of previous trauma, prior breast surgery (reduction mammoplasty, augmentation, lumpectomy), breast cancer (12%), inflammation, extensive physical activity, dehydration reported in some patients
- Mammography
  - Dilated vein—rope-like density, may have beaded appearance
  - Subcutaneous thickening parallel to palpable cord
- Ultrasound
  - Superficial, hypoechoic tubular structure
- Histology
  - Inflammation surrounding involved vessel
  - Involved veins recannulate.

Steatocystoma Multiplex

KEY FACTS

- Clinical
  - Autosomal dominant, but more common in males
  - Multiple cutaneous cysts appearing during adolescence and increasing progressively on anterior trunk, back, proximal extremities, external genitalia
  - Lesions are soft to firm and smooth, not usually larger than 2 cm in diameter; when incised, oily liquid is released.
  - Asymptomatic; may develop secondary inflammatory changes
  - Other possible diagnoses in patients with multiple skin lesions: Gardner's syndrome, cutaneous metastases, lipomatosis, neurofibromatosis, multiple leiomyomas, glomangiomas, xanthomatosis, cysticercosis
- Mammography
  - Oil cysts bilaterally—reportedly larger number of cysts in axillary tail
- Histology
  - Thin squamous epithelial covering; epithelium may fold into cyst
  - Cyst may incorporate elements such as sebaceous glands.

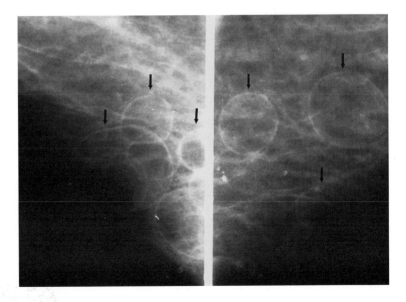

FIGURE 6-10
Steatocystoma multiplex. Multiple oil cysts bilaterally (*arrows*).

Inflammatory Carcinoma

KEY FACTS

- 1% of all breast cancers; definition of inflammatory carcinoma is debated: is the diagnosis dependent on the clinical findings of erythema, edema, and breast warmth, or is the diagnosis made on histologic sections demonstrating metastatic breast cancer in dermal lymphatics? Not all women with clinical findings suggestive of inflammatory carcinoma have involved dermal lymphatics, and not all patients with tumor emboli in the dermal lymphatics present with classic clinical signs.

- Clinical
  - Patients present with tender breast enlargement and firmness.
  - At presentation, differentiation from an acute inflammatory process (mastitis) may be difficult.
  - Erythema, edema (peau d'orange), and thickening of the skin, often involving the dependent portion of the breast, and breast warmth are the clinical findings required to make the diagnosis.
  - Approximately 80% of patients presenting with these findings have dermal lymphatic involvement on skin biopsy.
  - Approximately 4% of women with dermal lymphatic involvement do not demonstrate clinical signs associated with inflammatory carcinoma.
  - A discrete palpable mass may not be present.
  - Aggressive lesions having a poor prognosis: most patients die of disease within 2 years of diagnosis.

- Mammography
  - Affected breast is usually larger, less compressible, and denser than the contralateral normal breast.

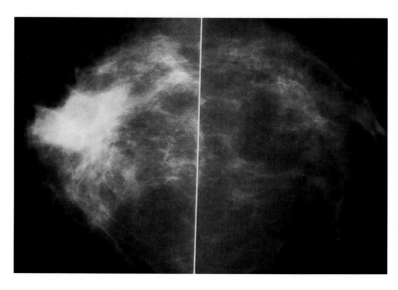

FIGURE 6-11
Inflammatory breast carcinoma. Diffuse increase in breast density, trabecular thickening, and architectural distortion. Right breast also appears smaller (contracted) compared to left. Edema, lymphatic obstruction, inflammation, trauma, and postlumpectomy or postradiation therapy changes would be in the differential. Invasive lobular carcinoma should also be included in the differential, along with inflammatory breast carcinoma.

- Skin and trabecular thickening are present, often without an identifiable dominant mass.

- On occasion, malignant calcifications can be seen scattered throughout the breast.

- Gross
  - Distinct tumor may not be identifiable; disease involves the breast diffusely.

- Histology
  - Dilated dermal lymphatics with tumor emboli
  - Associated inflammatory response in dermis surrounding vascular channels
  - Poorly differentiated invasive ductal carcinoma
  - Tumor emboli in vessels common

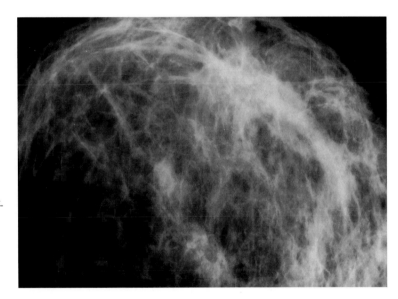

FIGURE 6-12
Inflammatory breast carcinoma. Diffuse trabecular thickening. Edema, lymphatic obstruction, inflammation, trauma, and postlumpectomy or postradiation therapy changes would be included in the differential.

Miscellaneous

- Skin necrosis
  - Reported secondary to anticoagulant therapy
  - Occurs in 0.1% of patients on coumadin (to be distinguished from cutaneous hemorrhage)
  - Presentation: obese woman with pain in an area of abundant subcutaneous fat 3 to 6 days after onset of treatment
  - Map-like ecchymosis of skin with halo of erythema
  - Progresses to bullous formation and skin necrosis
  - Etiology: thought to be direct toxicity of coumadin on endothelial cells
- Pyoderma gangrenosum
  - Mimics skin necrosis
  - May develop after minor surgery or trauma
  - Cutaneous ulcer: mucopurulent base, advancing purple discoloration and surrounding zone of erythema
  - Not an infectious process; possibly related to altered host immunity
- Candidal intertrigo
  - Inframammary area most commonly involved
  - Eroded, weepy lesion with scalloped borders and a red surrounding skin margin
- Herpes zoster
  - Virus lies dormant in dorsal root ganglia; distribution of cutaneous lesions follows sensory nerve distribution.
  - More common in winter
  - 10- to 20-day incubation period
  - 24-hour prodrome: fever, exanthem
  - 2- to 4-mm pink to red papules erupt and coalesce to form central 3- to 4-mm vesicle surrounded by red halo.
  - With leukocyte infiltration, the vesicles become turbid.
  - The lesion umbilicates, dies, and crusts over.
- Syphilis
  - Rare in developed countries
  - Primary and secondary cutaneous involvement of breast
  - Primary chancre heals in 2 to 6 weeks without treatment.
  - Secondary stage, on average 3 weeks after primary chancre: influenza-like presentation; diffuse lymphadenopathy; generalized rash (discrete lesions, sharply demarcated, coppery hue)
  - Early cutaneous manifestation of secondary syphilis includes macular or erythematous eruption on breast skin.

Nipple Changes Associated With Breast Cancer

KEY FACTS

- Nipple retraction
    - Underlying cancers can cause nipple skin thickening and retraction (nipple inversion).
    - Demonstration of lesion causing nipple retraction may require spot compression views. As the thickest part of the breast, the base may limit compression anteriorly. Also, given the convergence of ducts and possible nipple superimposition, the subareolar area may be ''busy.''

- Nipple ulceration
    - Related to Paget's disease
    - Advanced breast cancer extending out to involve surface of nipple

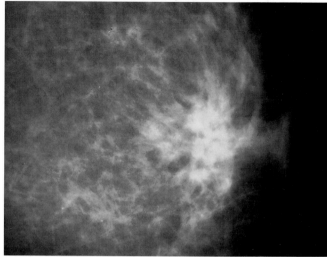

A

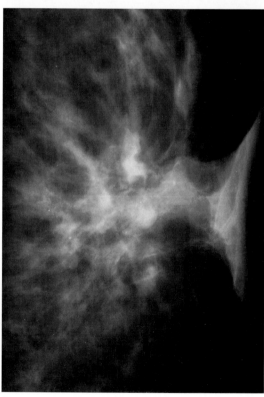

FIGURE 7-1
Infiltrating ductal carcinoma. (**A**) Architectural distortion associated with nipple skin thickening and possible retraction. (**B**) Subareolar micro-focus (0.1 mm) spot magnification view (1.8 ×). Architectural distortion, nipple skin thickening, and retraction are confirmed. A few scattered round, punctate microcalcifications are seen.

B

Dermatitis

KEY FACTS

- Clinical
  - Contact dermatitis: bacterial infection, irritation from clothes, soap, cosmetics, or unknown etiology
  - Differentiation from Paget's disease can be difficult.
  - Rapid time course, in contrast to slower development of Paget's
  - Nipple is not destroyed with dermatitis.
  - If the lesion involves the nipple only, it is more likely to be Paget's. If it involves both the nipple and areola, it is Paget's or (less likely) dermatitis. If it involves the areola and surrounding skin with no nipple involvement, it is not Paget's.

Nipple Adenoma

KEY FACTS

- Clinical
  - Nipple discharge most common complaint (65% to 70%)
  - Enlargement and induration, with possible ulceration of nipple.
  - Adenoma may protrude through duct orifice (friable, granulating mass).
  - Pain, itching or burning
- Mammography
  - Normal
  - Subareolar mass rare
- Ultrasound
  - Intraductal lesion extending to nipple
- Ductography
  - Filling defect extending to nipple (on cannulation of duct may see lesion protruding through duct orifice)
- Histology
  - Adenomatous proliferation of small tubules
  - May have associated epithelial proliferation

Hidradenitis Suppurativa

KEY FACTS

- Clinical
  - Chronic inflammatory process of the apocrine glands in areola (Montgomery's glands)
  - More common in women with chronic acne
  - Recurring nipple and areolar abscesses with associated draining sinuses, furuncles, and cellulitis
  - Superimposed bacterial infections can lead to deep central or subareolar abscesses.
- Mammography
  - Spiculated subareolar mass
  - Architectural distortion
  - Skin thickening
- Ultrasound
  - Complex mass, subareolar
  - May see connection of mass with skin (patent duct)—hypoechoic to anechoic tubular structure

Leiomyoma

KEY FACTS

- Superficial leiomyomata arise from smooth muscle—skin of areola.
- Vascular leiomyomata arise from smooth muscle—blood vessels. They are rare in breast tissue.

Paget's Disease

KEY FACTS

- Clinical
  - 1% to 5% of all breast carcinomas
  - Appearance of nipple varies depending on extent and stage of disease.
  - Initial: reddening of nipple and areola associated with pruritus
  - Progression: moist, scaling, eczematoid changes leading to ulceration and erosion of nipple
  - Approximately 50% of patients have a palpable mass.
  - Usually unilateral
  - 95% of patients have an underlying carcinoma (often poorly differentiated [comedo] ductal carcinoma in situ).
  - In situ carcinoma may be found in women with no palpable abnormality.
  - Occasionally intraductal papillomas protrude onto the nipple surface, producing a weeping, red lesion, so that Paget's comes into the differential. A palpable mass, however, is usually identified with papillomas (unlike Paget's).

- Mammography
  - Normal in many patients
  - Nipple and areolar thickening
  - Nipple calcifications
  - Subareolar mass

- Histology
  - Large cells (Paget's cells) with abundant pale cytoplasm and large nuclei with prominent nucleoli (adenocarcinoma cells) on the surface epithelium of the nipple
  - Cells may have melanin pigment (phagocytosis).

BIBLIOGRAPHY

Fornage BD, Faroux MJ, Pluot M, Gogomoletz W. Nipple adenoma simulating carcinoma: misleading clinical, mammographic, sonographic and cytologic findings. J Ultrasound Med 1991;10:55–57

Gilula LA, Destouet JM, Monsees B. Nipple simulating a breast mass on a mammogram. Radiology 1989;170:272

Haagensen CD. Paget's carcinoma of the breast. In Diseases of the breast, 3d ed. Philadelphia, WB Saunders, 1986, pp 758–781

Ikeda DM, Helvie MA, Frank TS, Chaper KL, Andersson IT. Paget disease of the nipple: radiologic–pathologic correlation. Radiology 1993;189:89–94

Page DL, Anderson TJ. Diagnostic histopathology of the breast. Edinburgh, Churchill Livingstone, 1987.

Tabár L, Dean PB. Teaching atlas of mammography. New York, Thieme Verlag, 1985.

Tavassoli FA. Pathology of the breast. New York, Elsevier, 1992.

Breast Imaging Companion
by Gilda Cardenosa
Lippincott-Raven Publishers, Philadelphia © 1997

Chapter 8

MAJOR SUBAREOLAR DUCTS

Normal Anatomy

KEY FACTS

- Although gross ductal anatomy has been debated, few studies have been done to evaluate breast ducts and ductal anatomy in normal and diseased states.
- The number of major ducts varies (estimates range from eight to 20).
- The branching pattern and distribution of ducts in the breast vary among women and in individual women during the course of their lifetime.
- The concept of "lobes," "segments," and "quadrants" in the breast, as though these can be defined anatomically, must be reevaluated. It is probably impossible to isolate a single duct as defining a lobe, segment, or quadrant. Ducts do not delineate specific anatomic areas in the breast: they overlap and can have widely divergent courses.
- The collecting duct is the portion of duct connecting the ductal orifice on the nipple to the lactiferous sinus.
- Lactiferous sinuses, in turn, connect to major subareolar ducts.
- The major subareolar ducts divide into a variable number of subsegmental ducts.
- Subsegmental ducts, in turn, divide into a variable number of terminal duct lobular units.
- Unless dilated or calcified, ducts are usually not seen on mammography. They may be seen for variable lengths on ultrasound as tubular structures converging on the subareolar area.
- On ductograms, normal ducts are variable in branching and distribution (caliber 1 to 2 mm).
- A single, contiguous layer of epithelial cells lines the duct lumen; basilar, intermittent, myoepithelial cells are interposed variably at the base of the epithelial cells.
- Elastic tissue surrounds the major and subsegmental ducts in the breast.

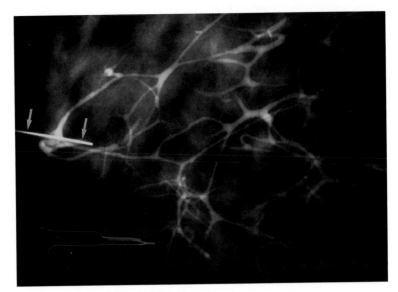

FIGURE 8-1
Normal duct (1.6 ×) on ductography. Duct branching and tissue distribution are variable. Normal caliber, 1 to 2 mm. A 30-G sialography cannula (*arrows*) in the duct can serve as a reference point for normal ductal caliber.

Duct Ectasia

KEY FACTS

- Clinical
  - Nipple discharge (thick, milky)
  - Nipple retraction
  - Pain and tenderness, often localized to subareolar area
  - Mass in subareolar area
  - Different terms have been used, including periductal mastitis and (erroneously) plasma cell mastitis, comedomastitis, and mastitis obliterans.

- Mammography
  - Many women have subareolar ductal prominence or dilatation mammographically; few, however, are symptomatic.
  - Dilated subareolar ducts may require subareolar spot compression views to exclude an underlying mass.
  - Coarse, smooth-bordered, rod-like, cigar-shaped calcifications (secretory) point toward the nipple and involve both breasts diffusely. If the calcifications form periductally (as opposed to intraductally), a central lucency is seen in the coarse, linear calcifications.
  - In the end stage, fibrosis may be seen in the subareolar area with coarse calcifications.

- Ultrasound
  - Dilated subareolar ducts
  - May see periductal fibrosis as a hyperechoic area periductally

- Ductography
  - Opacified duct is dilated. No intraductal abnormality can be identified.

- Histology
  - Subareolar ductal dilatation, periductal inflammation (periductal mastitis), and fibrosis
  - Progressive fibrosis and thickening of duct walls leads to foreshortening and obliteration (mastitis obliterans) of the ducts.
  - Etiology and pathogenesis unknown
  - Suggested etiologic factors: dilatation of ducts with stasis of contents leading to an inflammatory response, or periductal inflammation leading to ductal disruption and dilatation
  - Pregnancy and lactation have been implicated, but duct ectasia has been reported in nulliparous women.

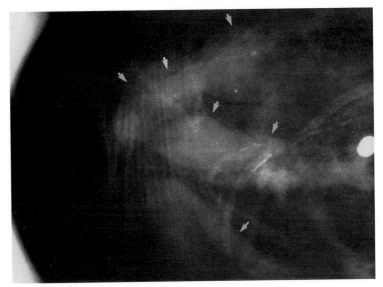

FIGURE 8-2
Duct ectasia. Subareolar spot compression demonstrates dilated, beaded, and tortuous subareolar ducts (*arrows*). On screening views, dilated subareolar ducts may appear mass-like. The subareolar area is relatively undercompressed in many women. If the base of the breast is thick, adequate compression anteriorly may be precluded. Spot compression views help elucidate ductal etiology.

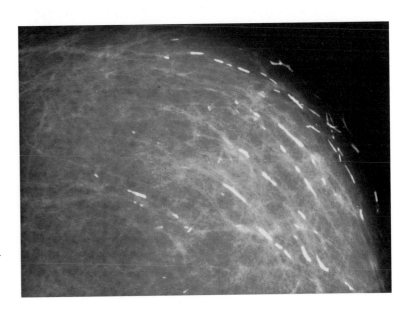

FIGURE 8-3
Benign ductal (secretory) calcifications. Dense, coarse, smooth border, commonly diffuse and bilateral, pointing toward the nipple.

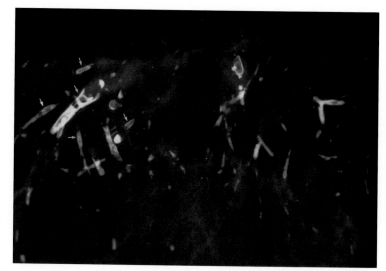

FIGURE 8-4

Benign ductal (secretory) calcifications. Dense, coarse, and smooth border (the ductal epithelium is flattened or denuded and there is no active epithelial proliferation, so the calcifications formed have smooth borders). If calcifications form periductally rather than intraductally, a central lucency is seen (*arrows*).

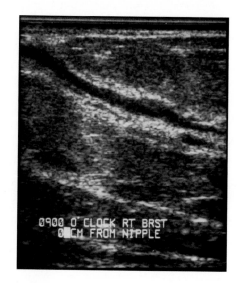

FIGURE 8-5

Periductal fibrosis seen as periductal hyperechogenicity on ultrasound.

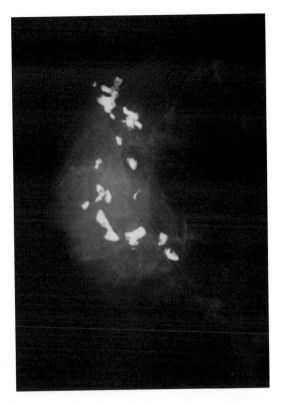

FIGURE 8-6
End-stage duct ectasia. Fibrosis and
coarse calcifications in subareolar
area.

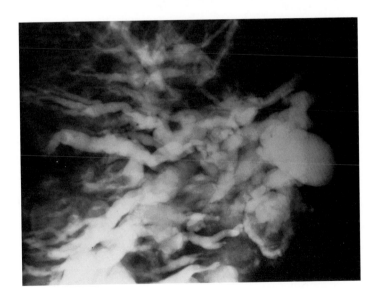

FIGURE 8-7
Duct ectasia on ductography.

Solitary Papillomas

KEY FACTS

- Clinical
  - Spontaneous nipple discharge (clear, serous, bloody)
  - Not usually palpable
  - Trigger point (Haagensen): pressure applied over the area of the papilloma reliably elicits discharge
  - Associated with slight increase in relative risk of breast cancer (1.5 to 2 ×)
- Mammography
  - Normal in most patients
  - Single dilated duct
  - Coarse or punctate calcifications, often in a subareolar location
- Ultrasound
  - Dilated duct with intraductal mass
  - Solid, homogeneously hypoechoic mass
- Ductography
  - Complete obstruction of duct by lesion (meniscus seen at point of obstruction)
  - Intraluminal filling defect
  - Ductal wall irregularity (sessile like papilloma)
  - Expansion and apparent distortion of duct
  - Segment of duct between lesion and nipple usually dilated
- Gross
  - Friable, soft lesion in duct (can be lost during specimen processing, so let the pathologist know you think a papilloma may be present so that the specimen is processed with extra care)
- Histology
  - Epithelial and myoepithelial cells (as arranged in normal ducts) capping fibrovascular core
  - Hyperplasia, atypical hyperplasia, and ductal carcinoma in situ may affect the epithelial elements of the papilloma.

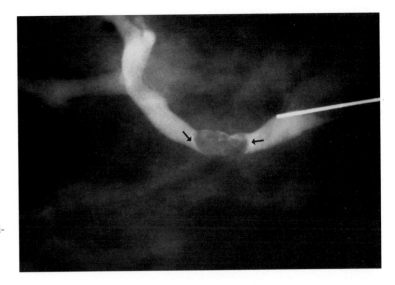

FIGURE 8-8
Solitary papilloma producing filling defect on ductogram. Note ductal caliber (relative to cannula) and menisci at leading edges of papilloma (*arrows*).

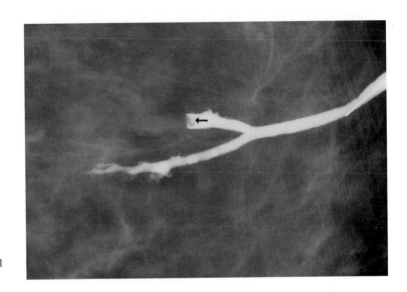

FIGURE 8-9
Solitary papilloma producing ductal obstruction on ductogram (*arrow*).

Papillary Carcinoma

KEY FACTS

- 1% to 2% of all breast cancers; older patients (mean age 63 to 67); higher incidence reported among African-American women

- Clinical
  - Nipple discharge (22% to 34%)
  - Nipple retraction or deviation
  - Palpable, often large, lobulated, circumscribed mass, commonly in the subareolar area (90%)
  - The lesion may protrude, stretching overlying skin and causing erythema and sometimes ulceration.
  - Estrogen receptor–positive; slow growth rate

- Mammography
  - Large, well-circumscribed masses (may be macrolobulated) in subareolar area
  - Benign-appearing calcifications may be associated with the mass.
  - Single or multiple clusters of calcifications—pleomorphic, linear, branching, coarse, round

- Ultrasound
  - Complex cystic mass (although seemingly developing in a cyst, these are thought to develop in ducts) with a variable solid component
  - Solid components may predominate with no associated fluid collection.

- Gross
  - Soft, friable tumors
  - Hemorrhagic fluid may be found in dilated duct or cyst.

- Histology
  - Noninvasive and invasive variants
  - Intraductal carcinoma variants (noninvasive papillary carcinomas) in the absence of stromal or vascular invasion
  - Most papillary carcinomas are found in a dilated duct (less commonly as an intracystic lesion).
  - No myoepithelial cells are present in papillary processes (present in benign papillary processes).
  - Epithelial cells in papillary carcinomas demonstrate carcinoembryonic antigen reactivity in 85% and may contain neurosecretory-type cytoplasmic granules, features not found in benign papillomas.
  - Stromal invasion in a small proportion of women
  - Well-differentiated, cribriform, micropapillary-type ductal carcinoma in situ can be found in adjacent tissue.

Breast Imaging Companion
by Gilda Cardenosa
Lippincott-Raven Publishers, Philadelphia © 1997

Chapter 9

TERMINAL DUCTS

Normal Anatomy

KEY FACTS

- The terminal duct lobular unit (TDLU) is divided arbitrarily into terminal duct and lobular segments.
- The terminal duct is divided into extralobular and intralobular segments.
- The two cell layers described for major subareolar and subsegmental ducts are also found in the terminal duct: a contiguous epithelial cell layer lining the lumen of the ducts and a discontinuous, basilar, myoepithelial cell layer.
- Unlike the major subareolar and subsegmental ducts, terminal ducts are not surrounded by elastic tissue.
- The stroma surrounding TDLUs is distinct: loose, rich in capillaries, and cellular.
- Most ductal breast cancers are thought to arise in the extralobular segment of the terminal duct.

Ductal Hyperplasia

KEY FACTS

- Hyperplasia refers to cellular proliferation only.

- Hyperplasia is present when there are more than two cell layers (normal) lining a duct. In more severe cases, ducts are usually distended by the proliferating cells.

- Mild, moderate, severe, and atypical are terms used by pathologists to qualify ductal hyperplasia.

- Some atypical ductal hyperplasias and borderline lesions (ie, atypical ductal hyperplasia versus well-differentiated ductal carcinoma in situ [DCIS]) may present a challenge to pathologists. Variation has been described among pathologists in their classification of these lesions.

- A slightly higher relative risk (1.5 to 2 ×) for the development of breast cancer has been described in women with mild to moderate ductal hyperplasia.

- A moderate relative risk (5 ×) for breast cancer development has been described in women with atypical ductal hyperplasia; this risk increases (10 to 11 ×) if atypical ductal hyperplasia is diagnosed in women with a positive family history (first-degree relative) of breast cancer.

- Ductal hyperplasia is thought to be a common component of fibrocystic change. It may be in a constant state of flux. In some women, atypical ductal hyperplasia and well-differentiated DCIS are probably also reversible.

- It has been proposed that in some women there is progression (evolution) from ductal hyperplasia to atypical ductal hyperplasia to DCIS and eventually to invasive ductal carcinoma. This theory, however, remains unproven and controversial. Some suggest that this evolution may be applicable to some types of breast cancers only (ie, to well-differentiated DCIS but not to poorly differentiated DCIS).

- Ductal hyperplasia can be an incidental finding in biopsies done for clinical or mammographic findings. In 40% to 50% of patients, the mammographic findings (most commonly microcalcifications) are directly correlated with the area of hyperplasia.

- Ductal distention and cellular proliferation characterize the ductal hyperplasias and DCIS. Microscopic evaluation of the cells, their nuclei, and proliferative patterns is needed to distinguish between these processes. It is not surprising that, morphologically, the calcifications that develop in association with ductal hyperplasia, atypical ductal hyperplasia, and well-differentiated DCIS are similar mammographically. Linear, casting-type calcifications remain the hallmark of poorly differentiated DCIS and are usually distinctive enough so as not to be confused with ductal hyperplasia, atypical ductal hyperplasia, or well-differentiated DCIS-type calcifications. Unfortunately, linear calcifications are seen in up to 22% of patients with well-differentiated DCIS.

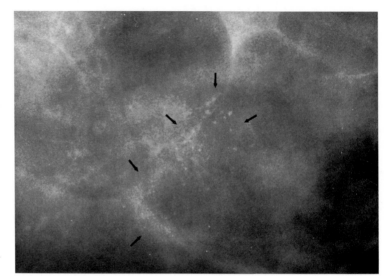

FIGURE 9-1

Atypical ductal hyperplasia. Cluster of punctate, irregular microcalcifications (*arrows*). Well-differentiated (low nuclear grade) ductal carcinoma in situ, hyperplasia, sclerosing adenosis, fibroadenoma, and multiple papillomas would be in the differential.

Multiple (Peripheral) Papillomas

KEY FACTS

- Clinical

  - Usually asymptomatic, diagnosed on biopsies done for mammographic findings

  - Spontaneous nipple discharge in approximately 20% of patients

  - Possible marker lesion for increased breast cancer risk, but no long-term epidemiologic studies have been done to confirm this

  - Develop in terminal duct (hence the "peripheral papilloma" designation)—may explain why some of these lesions appear as "intracystic" (in contrast to solitary papillomas, which, although occurring within dilated ducts, are not commonly intracystic). We postulate that as the papillomas develop, they obstruct the TDLU, with resultant accumulation of fluid, effacement of acini, and cyst formation.

- Mammography

  - Multiple, small, well-circumscribed or partially circumscribed masses

  - Cluster or multiple clusters of punctate, pleomorphic calcifications; no linear or casting calcifications are usually seen, nor is there significant ductal orientation within the calcification clusters

  - Findings (either masses or microcalcifications) may be bilateral.

- Ultrasound

  - Solid, homogeneously hypoechoic mass or masses

  - Intracystic mass

- Histology

  - Indistinguishable from solitary papillomas

  - Two cell layers: contiguous epithelial cell layer (contiguous with ductal epithelium) and discontinuous myoepithelial, basilar layer

  - Fibrovascular core

  - In up to 43% of our patients, atypical ductal hyperplasia, DCIS (well- to moderately differentiated), or lobular neoplasia is seen in the parenchyma adjacent to multiple papillomas. The presence of these proliferative changes may justify the consideration of these lesions as breast cancer risk marker lesions.

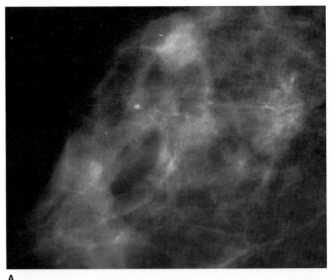

A

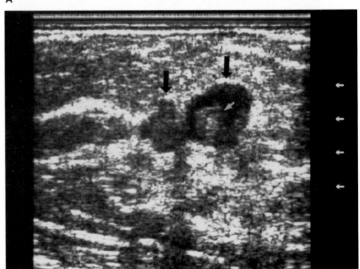

FIGURE 9-2

Multiple papillomas. (**A**) Cluster of masses with ill-defined margins. (**B**) Irregular, lobulated mass (*black arrows*). Part of the soft-tissue component is intracystic (*white arrow*).

B

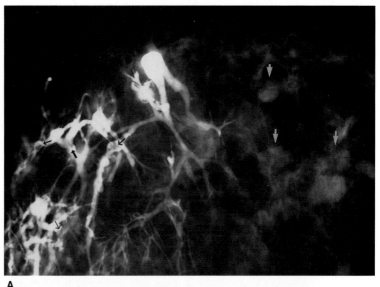

A

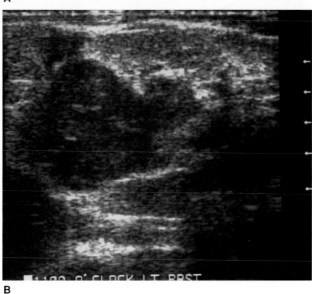

FIGURE 9-3
(**A**) Multiple papillomas and papillary carcinomas. Multiple masses (*white arrows*) with ill-defined margins in the medial portion of the breast. Multiple filling defects (*black arrows*) and duct wall irregularity on ductography, lateral duct. (**B**) Lobulated, hypoechoic mass with some posterior acoustic enhancement.

B

Radial Scars—Complex Sclerosing Lesions

KEY FACTS

- Clinical
    - Not related to previous trauma or surgery (don't let the word "scar" mislead you); etiology unknown
    - Controversial significance: benign, high-risk marker, or premalignant? In up to 30% to 40% of patients, reported to contain or be associated with areas of atypical ductal hyperplasia, DCIS (well-to moderately differentiated), lobular neoplasia, and tubular carcinoma
    - Radial scars measure 1 to 9 mm; common histologically but not readily apparent mammographically
    - Complex sclerosing lesions are larger than 10 mm; may be incidental finding in biopsies done for unrelated clinical or mammographic findings, but can be suspected in some women after appropriate mammographic work-up
    - Unclear if the only difference between radial scars and complex sclerosing lesions is size
    - Not usually palpable

- Mammography
    - Spiculated lesion characterized by a central fatty area and long, thin radiating spicules
    - Differential appearance between views: well seen in one projection, harder to identify in orthogonal view (planar lesions)
    - Although the lesion may be large, there is usually no correlative palpable abnormality.
    - When suspected on mammography, excisional biopsy with deferment of frozen section is recommended. These can be difficult lesions to diagnose (on histology, the differential diagnosis includes tubular carcinoma and sclerosing adenosis).
    - When we suspect a complex sclerosing lesion, we recommend excisional biopsy (as opposed to core biopsy) for two reasons. First, the pathologist may have a difficult time making a precise diagnosis. Second, even if the pathologist can make a diagnosis on a core biopsy, the high incidence of associated proliferative changes with and without atypia, lobular neoplasia, and tubular carcinoma is such that we feel these lesions are best excised.
    - If we do a core biopsy on a woman with a spiculated mass and the histologic diagnosis is that of radial scar or complex sclerosing lesion (or if the pathologist says these lesions cannot be excluded), we recommend excisional biopsy after preoperative wire localization.

- Ultrasound
    - Patients do not usually have an ultrasound (spiculated mass mammographically; no clinical symptoms).
    - In the few patients evaluated with ultrasound, we have seen an irregular area of shadowing not associated with a discrete mass.

- Histology
  - Central fibroelastotic core from which spicules of proliferating epithelial elements arise; epithelial proliferation without atypia (epithelial hyperplasia, sclerosing adenosis), with atypia (atypical ductal hyperplasia, lobular neoplasia) and well- to intermediately differentiated DCIS
  - Tubular carcinomas have been reported in association with complex sclerosing lesions.

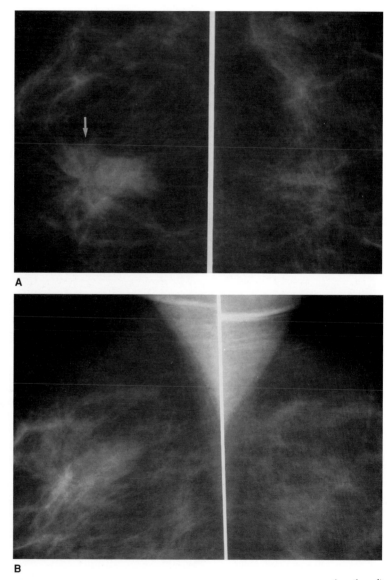

FIGURE 9-4
Complex sclerosing lesion. (A) Right and left craniocaudal (CC) views back to back. Spiculated mass (*arrow*) with central lucency and associated architectural distortion, medial right breast. (B) Right and left mediolateral oblique (MLO) views back to back. Architectural distortion less conspicuous than on CC view, right breast superiorly.

A

B

(continued)

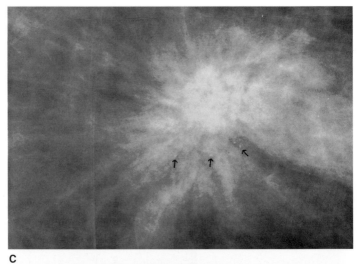

C

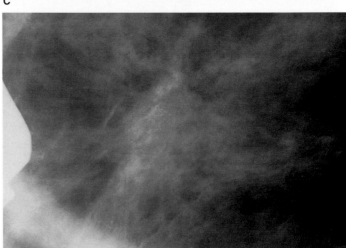

D

FIGURE 9-4 (CONTINUED)
(**C**) Magnified (1.8 ×) CC view demonstrates spiculated mass with some
central lucency, scattered punctate calcifications (*arrows*), and long radiating spicules. On physical examination, no mass could be palpated in
the expected location of this lesion.
(**D**) Magnified (1.8 ×) MLO view.
Although there is architectural distortion, the overall appearance of the
mass is different from that seen on
the CC view. (**E**) Specimen radiograph. Spiculated mass with associated, scattered, punctate calcifications.

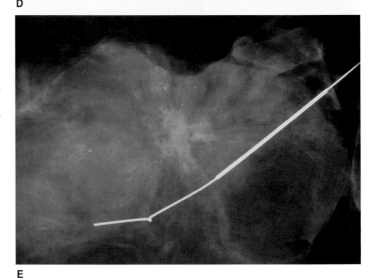

E

Ductal Adenoma

KEY FACTS

- Clinical
  - Mass
  - Not associated with nipple discharge

- Mammography
  - Mass, well- to partially defined margins
  - Microcalcifications

- Histology
  - Well-defined glandular proliferation (epithelial and myoepithelial cells)
  - May be variants of sclerosing papillomas
  - Some lesions also include features of complex sclerosing lesions and fibrosing tubular adenomas.

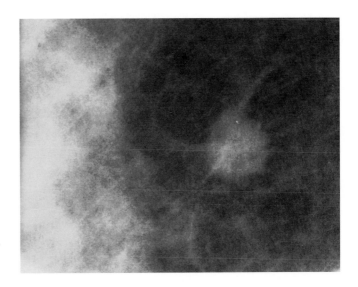

FIGURE 9-5
Ductal adenoma. Micro-focus spot magnification view (1.8 ×) of small mass with ill-defined margins.

Ductal Carcinoma in Situ (DCIS)

KEY FACTS

- Before the advent of high-quality mammographic studies and the ability to detect microcalcifications, DCIS was considered a rare type of breast cancer. It now constitutes 22% to 45% of all breast cancers diagnosed mammographically.

- Based on biologic markers, three-dimensional studies, and histology, as well as mammographic and clinical presentation, DCIS is a heterogeneous disease.

- Clinical
  - Most patients are asymptomatic.
  - They may, however, present with a palpable mass, spontaneous nipple discharge, or Paget's disease.

- Mammography
  - Clusters of pleomorphic, ductally oriented microcalcifications
  - Less commonly, DCIS can produce a mass with ill-defined or lobulated borders (not usually spiculated), which may or may not have associated malignant-type calcifications.
  - Architectural distortion

- Ultrasound
  - High specular echoes (calcifications)
  - Associated soft-tissue component and architectural distortion may reflect dilated ducts or the presence of an invasive component.

- Gross
  - Cut surface through an area of poorly differentiated (comedo) DCIS may be associated with the presence of comedos, the necrotic contents of abnormal ducts.
  - No gross abnormality is usually evident with well- to intermediately differentiated DCIS.

- Histology
  - Based on nuclear and architectural features, subclassified into well-differentiated, (low nuclear grade, cribriform, micropapillary, solid, small cell), intermediately differentiated, or poorly differentiated (high nuclear grade, comedo, large cell)

WELL-DIFFERENTIATED DCIS (LOW NUCLEAR GRADE)

- Ductal distention with monomorphic cellular proliferation creating cribriform spaces (punched out) or micropapillary processes; solid growth present in some
- Necrosis uncommon
- Calcifications develop in secretions.
- Monomorphic nuclei, small or absent nucleoli
- Mitotic figures rare

- No individual cell necrosis, no autophagocytosis
- Cellular polarization
- Multifocal origin and growth (almost 50% of patients)
- Punctate, round calcifications; multifocal
- Microcalcifications seen mammographically may not be intimately associated with histologic disease. Mammographically, we underestimate the extent of disease found histologically.
- Approximately 47% of lesions calcify.

INTERMEDIATELY DIFFERENTIATED DCIS

- Moderately differentiated nuclei
- Polarization of cells
- Linearly oriented, punctate microcalcifications—pleomorphic, mixture of round and linear microcalcifications

POORLY DIFFERENTIATED DCIS (HIGH NUCLEAR GRADE)

- Ductal distention with pleomorphic cellular proliferation circumferentially encroaching the duct lumen
- Central necrosis generally present
- Distended ducts with periductal fibrosis and lymphocytes
- Pleomorphic nuclei with multiple nucleoli
- Mitotic figures
- Individual cell necrosis and autophagocytosis
- No true cellular polarization
- Linearly oriented, pleomorphic microcalcifications; may extend to subareolar area
- Close association between microcalcifications seen mammographically and extent of disease found histologically
- Approximately 90% of lesions calcify.

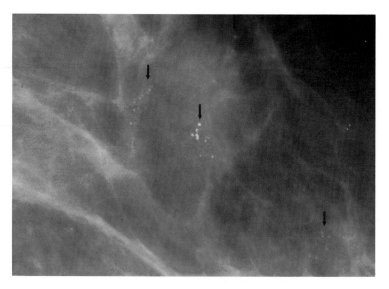

FIGURE 9-6

Well-differentiated (low nuclear grade) ductal carcinoma in situ (DCIS). Micro-focus spot magnification view (1.8 ×) demonstrates multiple clusters of punctate (mixed round and irregular) calcifications with variable density. Intervening portions of breast tissue may be normal or demonstrate areas of ductal hyperplasia (mild, moderate, severe), atypical hyperplasia, or well-differentiated DCIS (with no associated microcalcifications). Mammography may underestimate the extent of disease.

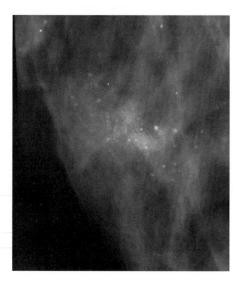

FIGURE 9-7

Well-differentiated (low nuclear grade) ductal carcinoma in situ. Micro-focus spot magnification view (1.8 ×) demonstrates cluster of irregular, round and punctate microcalcifications. This cluster of calcifications in the medial portion of the breast posteriorly developed compared with previous study.

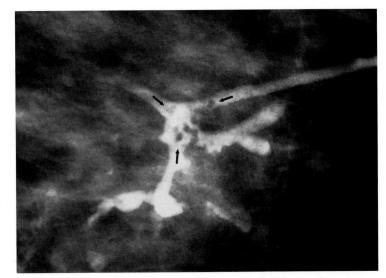

FIGURE 9-8
Well-differentiated (low nuclear grade) ductal carcinoma in situ. Ductal irregularity (*arrows*) on ductography. No microcalcifications or mass seen on preductogram mammogram. Patient presented with spontaneous nipple discharge (serosanguineous).

FIGURE 9-9
Poorly differentiated (high nuclear grade) ductal carcinoma in situ (DCIS). Linear (casting) calcifications. Irregular border and clefts within calcifications are common. Morphology better appreciated on micro-focus spot magnification view (1.8 ×). Density of calcifications variable. Mammography fairly accurate in demonstrating the extent of poorly differentiated DCIS (where we see calcifications is where the pathologist finds DCIS).

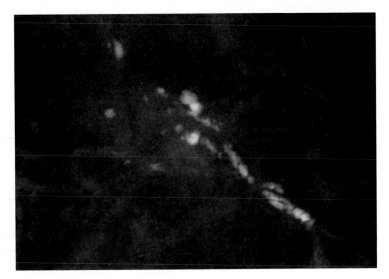

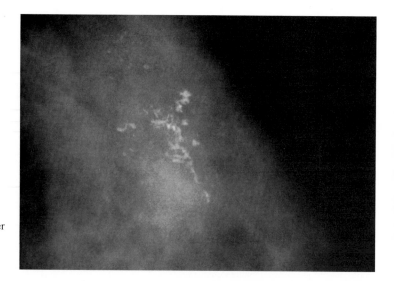

FIGURE 9-10
Poorly differentiated (high nuclear grade) ductal carcinoma in situ. Cluster of pleomorphic and linear calcifications on micro-focus spot magnification view (1.8 ×).

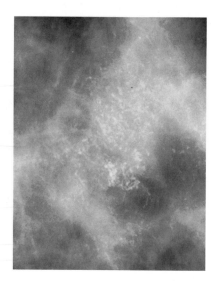

FIGURE 9-11
Poorly differentiated (high nuclear grade) ductal carcinoma in situ. Cluster of pleomorphic, predominantly linear calcifications. Low density. Many of these calcifications could not be seen on screening view. Micro-focus spot magnification useful in evaluating calcification morphology, finding additional calcifications within a given cluster, and demonstrating additional calcification clusters.

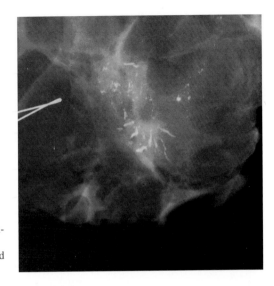

FIGURE 9-12
Poorly differentiated (high nuclear grade) ductal carcinoma in situ. Specimen radiograph (with compression and 1.6 × magnification). Linear and punctate microcalcifications.

FIGURE 9-13
Poorly differentiated (high nuclear grade) ductal carcinoma in situ (DCIS). Screening studies 1 year apart photographed back to back for comparison. Irregular mass (*arrow*) developed in 1 year. Distended ducts in aggregate and associated periductal inflammation probably explain the presentation of DCIS as a mass (in our material, less than 5% of DCIS).

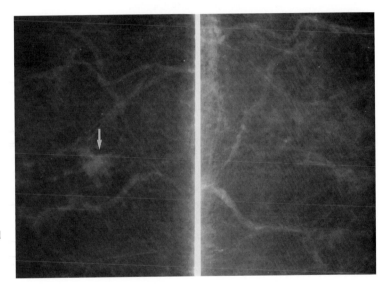

Invasive Ductal Carcinoma Not Otherwise Specified (NOS)

KEY FACTS

- Most common type of breast cancer (constitutes approximately 65% to 75% of all breast cancers)—no specific histologic findings or patterns present to subclassify as a "special" breast cancer type

- Clinical
  - Palpable mass
  - Focal breast tenderness
  - Nipple discharge
  - Skin retraction or ulceration in women with advanced disease

- Mammography
  - Spiculated mass
  - Round, well-defined or partially defined mass. These types of masses are most commonly associated with some of the "special" breast cancer types, but because NOS is so common, the most common histologic finding in women with well-defined or partially defined masses is invasive ductal carcinoma NOS.
  - Architectural distortion (isolated or associated with a mass)
  - Malignant-type calcifications can be seen with any of the above findings. When malignant calcifications are associated with a soft-tissue component, the patient usually has a combination of invasive ductal carcinoma and DCIS. The presence of an extensive intraductal component (EIC) may be of prognostic significance. The rate of local recurrence after conservative treatment is reportedly higher in women with EIC, particularly younger women ages 40 to 49. This may be related to the presence of residual disease in the breast. It is important to alert the surgeon and pathologist when EIC is suspected mammographically.

how can this be suspected mammographically?

- Ultrasound
  - Hypoechoic mass; marked hypoechogenicity common
  - Spiculation
  - Microlobulated margins
  - Vertical orientation (lesion is tall)
  - Angulated margins
  - Extension of tumor into distended ducts
- Histology
  - Variable architectural growth patterns (ie, tubule formation and appearance) and cellular morphology
  - Several grading systems are available. Most are modifications of the Bloom and Richardson grading system based on architectural growth patterns, nuclear morphology, and proliferative activity (mitotic count). All in situ lesions and invasive breast cancers measuring 1 cm or less in greatest diameter are considered minimal breast cancer.

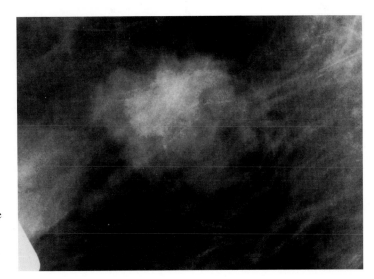

FIGURE 9-14
Invasive ductal carcinoma (not otherwise specified). Micro-focus spot magnification view (1.8 ×). Mass with lobulated, indistinct margins and no associated microcalcifications or satellite lesions.

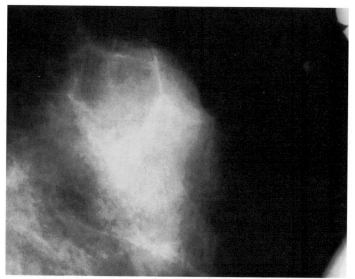

A

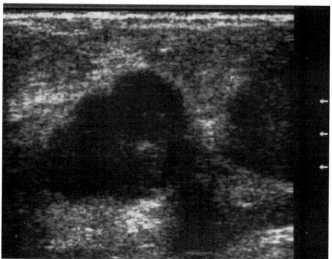

FIGURE 9-15
Invasive ductal carcinoma (not otherwise
specified). (**A**) Micro-focus spot magnification view (1.8 ×). Palpable mass with indistinct margins and no associated microcalcifications. (**B**) Hypoechoic mass with
heterogeneous echo texture, and vertical
orientation (taller than wide).

B

FIGURE 9-16

Invasive ductal carcinoma (not otherwise specified). Micro-focus spot magnification view (1.6 ×). Spiculated mass, low density with associated microcalcifications (ductal carcinoma in situ on histology). Given the presence of central fat and long spicules, postoperative changes (fat necrosis) and a complex sclerosing lesion should be included in the differential. Patient had no prior history of surgery or trauma. Although no discrete mass could be palpated, the entire area was hard (indurated), with some subtle dimpling when the arm was elevated (arguing against a complex sclerosing lesion). This underscores the importance of correlating the physical examination with the mammographic findings.

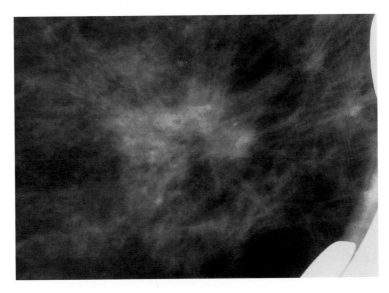

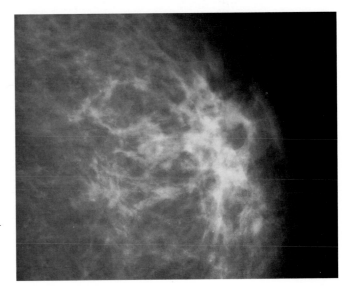

FIGURE 9-17

Invasive ductal carcinoma (not otherwise specified). Architectural distortion, left subareolar area with nipple retraction and thickening. Spot compression/magnification views can be done to confirm findings.

Tubular Carcinoma

KEY FACTS

- In pure form, less than 2% of all breast cancers; median age 44 to 49
- Clinical
  - Palpable mass, but most tubular carcinomas are diagnosed mammographically
  - Multicentric in up to 28% of patients, bilateral in 12% to 38%; family history of breast cancer in up to 40% of women diagnosed with tubular carcinoma
  - Pure lesions associated with excellent prognosis
- Mammography
  - Small spiculated mass
  - Indeterminate or malignant-type calcifications (may be apparent on magnification views only) within and beyond the spiculated mass
  - Look for satellite lesions, possibly bridging with the dominant spiculated mass; multicentricity is common.
- Gross
  - Tan, poorly circumscribed scirrhous mass; infiltrative
- Histology
  - Proliferation of angulated, oval, and elongated tubules lined by a single cell layer (no myoepithelial cells); cells may display apical snouts
  - Mitotic figures rare
  - Fibroblastic stroma may be dense and elastotic.
  - Calcification in up to 50% of lesions
  - Low-grade, well-differentiated, cribriform-type DCIS in up to 65% of patients
  - Lobular neoplasia (lobular carcinoma in situ) in close proximity in approximately 15%
  - Differentiating tubular carcinomas from sclerosing adenosis and complex sclerosing lesions (radial scars) can be difficult, particularly on frozen sections.

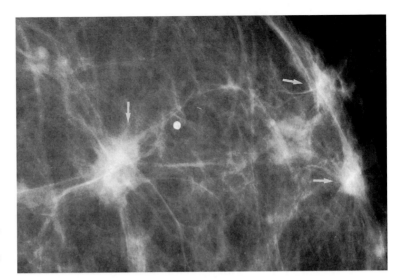

FIGURE 9-18
Tubular carcinoma. Micro-focus spot magnification view (1.8 ×) demonstrates dominant spiculated mass and two additional spiculated masses (*arrows*) not appreciated on screening views. Bridging between small spiculated masses is common with tubular carcinomas.

Mucinous Carcinoma

KEY FACTS

- 2% of all breast cancers; can occur at all ages, but more common in older women (1% in women less than age 35 and 7% in women older than 75)
- Clinical
  - Mass lesion; palpatory "swish" sign described by Halstead rare
  - Slow growth rate
  - Good short-term prognosis for pure lesions, but systemic recurrences more than 10 years after initial treatment have been reported
  - Prognosis of mixed lesions (mucinous and invasive NOS components) determined by the characteristics of the invasive component
  - Commonly diploid, estrogen receptor positive
  - Mucin embolization a rare complication
- Mammography
  - Round mass; borders may be well defined to obscured
- Ultrasound
  - Well-circumscribed, hypoechoic, homogeneous (may be heterogeneous) mass
  - Posterior acoustic enhancement a prominent feature in some women
- Gross
  - Glistening cut surface, soft consistency; well-defined, round, expansile lesions
- Histology
  - Aggregates of tumor cells surrounded completely by mucin and compartmentalized by fibrovascular bands

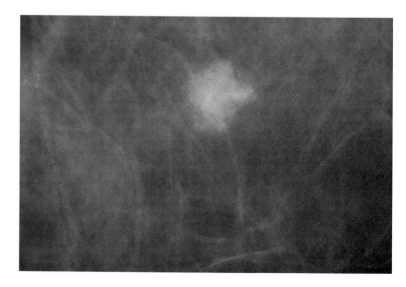

FIGURE 9-19
Mucinous carcinoma. Round mass.

- Cellularity of aggregates varies from a few to large clumps of malignant cells floating in mucin.
- Cells contain little intracellular mucin.
- Necrosis uncommon
- Well-differentiated DCIS (cribriform) may be found in adjacent breast tissue, but DCIS is not a prominent component of these lesions.

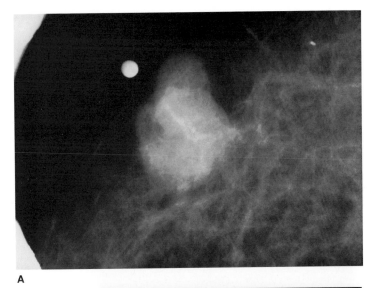

A

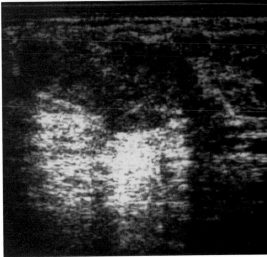

B

FIGURE 9-20
Mucinous carcinoma. (**A**) Spot compression. Palpable well-defined, lobulated mass. (**B**) Hypoechoic mass with posterior acoustic enhancement.

Medullary Carcinoma

KEY FACTS

- 5% to 7% of all breast cancers. The reported variation in frequency may be due to differences in definition criteria used by pathologists; however, with strict adherence to diagnostic histologic criteria, this tumor may not be as common as reported previously.

- More common in younger women (11% of all breast cancers in women younger than age 35), rare in elderly patients

- Clinical
  - Circumscribed, mobile mass lesion (given the young age of many patients, may be mistaken for a fibroadenoma)
  - Fast growth rate, high thymidine labeling
  - Usually aneuploid, estrogen receptor negative
  - Locally aggressive. Despite aggressive histologic features, the prognosis of pure medullary carcinomas is better than that seen with infiltrating ductal carcinomas (NOS).
  - If fatal, death usually occurs within 5 years of diagnosis.

- Mammography
  - Round mass, ill-defined borders

- Ultrasound
  - Solid, homogeneously hypoechoic round mass

- Gross
  - Well-defined, round, expansile lesion; soft in consistency
  - May have associated areas of hemorrhage or necrosis

- Histology
  - Strict adherence to histologic criteria critical for diagnostic accuracy
  - Intense lymphoplasmacytic reaction around and within tumor
  - Syncytial, solid, sheet-like growth pattern of medium to large anaplastic cells, high mitotic rate
  - Gross and microscopic necrosis, but calcification uncommon
  - Plasma cells associated with these tumors produce IgA, in contrast to IgG-producing plasma cells seen in infiltrating ductal carcinoma (NOS).
  - In situ component rare

ATYPICAL MEDULLARY CARCINOMAS

- Lesions with a syncytial growth pattern of anaplastic cells having foci of infiltrating ductal carcinoma (NOS), dense fibrosis, or fibrous bands and lacking a significant lymphoplasmacytic reaction

- Atypical medullary carcinomas do not have the good prognosis of pure medullary carcinomas; prognosis is similar to that of infiltrating ductal carcinomas (NOS). Strict adherence to diagnostic criteria is critical.

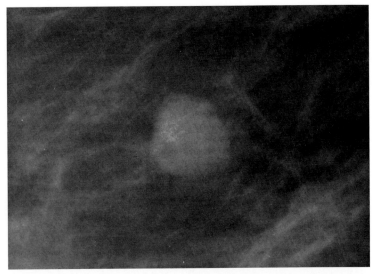

A

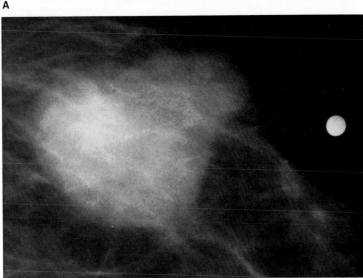

B

FIGURE 9-21
Medullary carcinoma. (**A**) Well-defined mass. (**B**) One year later, the mass is significantly larger and is now lobulated and palpable. This tumor is locally aggressive.

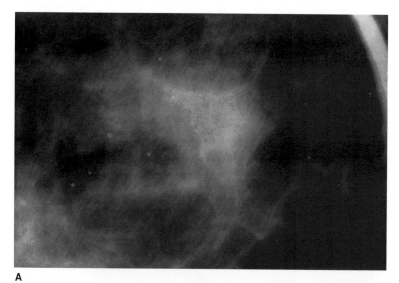

A

B

FIGURE 9-22
Atypical medullary carcinoma. (**A**) Micro-focus spot magnification view (1.8 ×). Ill-defined mass. (**B**) Hypoechoic mass. Medullary carcinomas are often markedly hypoechoic.

Invasive Cribriform Carcinoma

KEY FACTS

- Clinical
  - 1.7% to 3.5% of all breast cancers
  - Excellent prognosis

- Mammography
  - Well- to ill-defined mass
  - Microcalcifications may be present.

- Histology
  - Stromal invasion
  - Same cribriform arrangement seen in well-differentiated, cribriform DCIS
  - Approximately 25% of tumors have associated features of tubular carcinoma.
  - Well-differentiated, cribriform DCIS present in adjacent tissue (75%)
  - Differential includes tubular carcinoma, cribriform-type DCIS, and adenoid cystic carcinoma.

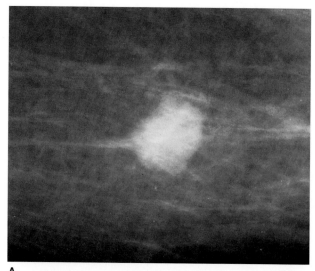

FIGURE 9-23
Invasive cribriform carcinoma. (**A**) Well-defined mass.
(**B**) Hypoechoic mass (taller than wide) with minimal
posterior acoustic shadowing.

BIBLIOGRAPHY

Adler DD, Helvie MA, Oberman HA, Ikeda DM, Bhan AO. Radial sclerosing lesion of the breast: mammographic features. Radiology 1990;176:737–740

Cardenosa G, Doudna C, Eklund GW. Mucinous (colloid) breast cancer: clinical and mammographic findings in 10 patients. AJR 1994;162:1077–1079

Cardenosa G, Eklund GW. Benign papillary neoplasms of the breast: mammographic findings. Radiology 1991;179:751–755

Ciatto S, Morrone D, Catarzi S, et al. Radial scars of the breast: review of 38 consecutive mammographic diagnoses. Radiology 1993;187:757–760

Elson BC, Helvie MA, Frank TS, Wilson TE, Adler DD. Tubular carcinoma of the breast: mode of presentation, mammographic appearance and frequency of nodal metastases. AJR 1993;161:1173–1176

Fechner RD, Mills SE. Breast pathology: benign proliferations, atypias and in situ carcinomas. Chicago, American Society of Clinical Pathologists, 1990.

Frouge C, Tristant H, Guinebretiere JM, et al. Mammographic lesions suggestive of radial scars: microscopic findings in 40 cases. Radiology 1995;195:623–625

Helvie MA, Hessler C, Frank TS, Ikeda DM. Atypical hyperplasia of the breast: mammographic appearance and histologic correlation. Radiology 1991;179:759–764

Helvie MA, Paramagul C, Oberman HA, Adler DD. Invasive tubular carcinoma: imaging features and clinical detection. Invest Radiol 1993;28:202–207

Holland R, Connolly JL, Gelman R, et al. The presence of an extensive intraductal component following a limited excision correlates with prominent residual disease in the remainder of the breast. J Clin Oncol 1990;8:113–118

Holland R, Hendriks JHCL, Verbeek ALM, Mravunac M, Stekhove JHS. Extent, distribution and mammographic/histological correlations of breast ductal carcinoma in situ. Lancet 1990;335:519–522

Ikeda DM. Andersson I. Ductal carcinoma in situ: atypical mammographic appearances. Radiology 1989;172:661–666

Leibman AJ, Lewis M, Kruse B. Tubular carcinoma of the breast: mammographic appearance. AJR 1993;160:263–265

Meyer JE, Amin E, Lindfors KK, Lipman JC, Stomper PC, Genest D. Medullary carcinoma of the breast: mammographic and US appearance. Radiology 1989;170:79–82

Millis RA, Eusebi V (eds). Ductal carcinoma in situ. Semin Diag Pathol 1994;11:167–235

Mitnick JS, Vasquez MF, Harris MN, Rosen DF. Differentiation of radial scar from scirrhous carcinoma of the breast: mammographic–pathologic correlation. Radiology 1989;173:697–700

Orel SG, Evers K, Yeh I-T, Troupin RH. Radial scar with microcalcifications: radiographic–pathologic correlation. Radiology 1992;183:479–482

Page DL, Anderson TJ. Diagnostic histopathology of the breast. Edinburgh, Churchill Livingstone, 1987.

Rosai J. Borderline epithelial lesions of the breast. Am J Surg Pathol 1991;15:209–221

Sickles EA. Breast masses: mammographic evaluation. Radiology 1989;173:297–303

Stomper PC, Cholewinski SP, Penetrante RB, Harlos JP, Tsangaris TN. Atypical ductal hyperplasia: frequency and mammographic and pathologic relationships in excisional biopsies guided with mammography and clinical examination. Radiology 1993;189:667–671

Stomper PC, Connolly JL. Ductal carcinoma in situ of the breast: correlation between mammographic calcification and tumor subtype. AJR 1992;159:483–485

Tabár L, Dean PB. Teaching atlas of mammography. New York, Thieme Verlag, 1985.

Tavassoli FA. Pathology of the breast. New York, Elsevier, 1992.

Wilson TE, Helvie MA, Oberman HA, et al. Pure and mixed mucinous carcinoma of the breast: pathologic basis for differences in mammographic appearance. AJR 1995;165:285–289

Breast Imaging Companion
by Gilda Cardenosa
Lippincott-Raven Publishers, Philadelphia © 1997

Chapter 10

LOBULES

Normal Anatomy

KEY FACTS

- Ducts terminate in blind-ending sacs: acini (grouped into lobules, like leaves on a branch).
- Lobules produce milk during pregnancy and lactation.
- Epithelial and myoepithelial cells are found in lobules.
- Unlike ductal elements, no elastic tissue is associated with lobules.
- On mammography, we cannot usually see lobules. On ultrasound, if a duct is traced back from the nipple, small hypoechoic mass-like areas can occasionally be seen, arranged around the duct; presumably these are acini.
- Round, sharply defined (pearl-like), high-density calcifications, either in tight clusters or scattered diffusely in both breasts, form in acini.
- On ductography, a contrast blush is seen in a few women, presumably representing filling of the acini with contrast. Why this contrast blush is not seen more often is unknown.

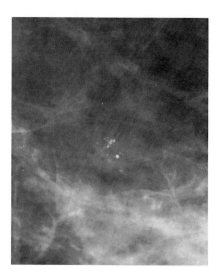

FIGURE 10-1
Lobular calcifications. Tight cluster of round calcifications.

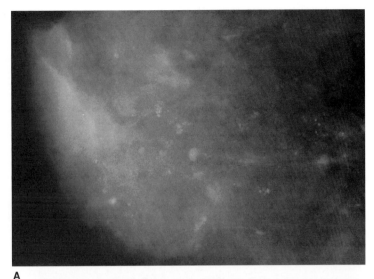

A

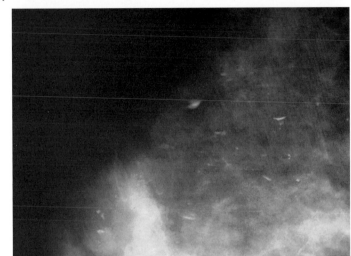

B

FIGURE 10-7
Milk of calcium. (**A**) Craniocaudal (CC)
view. Ill-defined, amorphous calcifications
scattered throughout breast parenchyma.
(**B**) 90° lateral view. Calcification layering
in dependent portion of microcysts. Sharp,
curvilinear ("teacup") calcifications. This
differential appearance between CC and
90° lateral views is the hallmark for milk
of calcium; benign calcifications require
no further evaluation or follow-up.

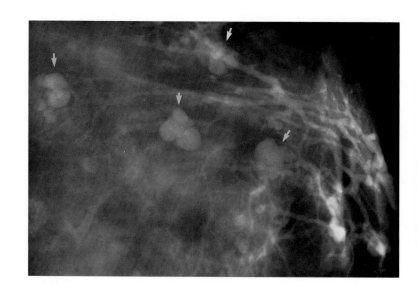

FIGURE 10-8
Cysts on ductography (*arrows*).

Galactocele

KEY FACTS

- Clinical
  - Cyst with inspissated milk
  - Palpable mass in pregnant or lactating patient; may be seen up to several years after lactation
  - May be multiple, uni- or bilateral
  - Diagnosed after aspiration
- Mammography
  - Well-circumscribed mass; density may be variable
  - Some may have mixed density with fat/fluid level on 90° lateral views.
- Ultrasound
  - Features of cyst: well-defined, anechoic mass
  - Solid mass with posterior acoustic enhancement
  - Shadowing

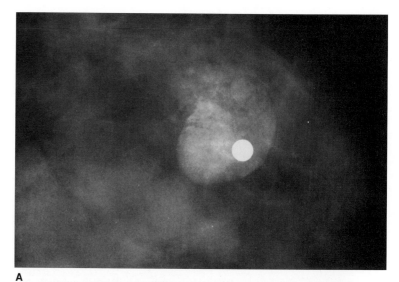

A

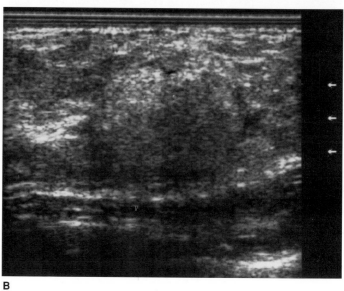

FIGURE 10-9
Galactocele. (**A**) Palpable mass (metallic BB). Fluid/fat level seen (variation in density of mass). (**B**) Lower portion of mass hypoechoic relative to upper portion (probable fluid/fluid level). Some shadowing is seen.

B

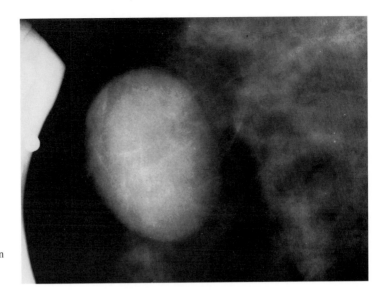

FIGURE 10-10
Galactocele. Well-circumscribed mass in women during lactation. Milky, thick fluid aspirated.

Juvenile Papillomatosis

KEY FACTS

- Clinical
  - Adolescents and young women (mean age 23)
  - Some reports suggest an increased incidence of breast cancer in women with juvenile papillomatosis and within the female members of the family.
  - No relation to parity, age at menarche, or use of birth-control pills
  - Painless, circumscribed, mobile mass
- Mammography
  - Not usually done because of patient age at time of presentation
- Gross
  - Well-circumscribed lesions
  - Multiple cysts (like Swiss cheese), some with papillary excrescences, dense stroma between cysts
- Histology
  - Multiple cysts
  - Well circumscribed but not encapsulated
  - Marked ductal hyperplasia (papillomatosis—bordering intraductal carcinoma), apocrine and nonapocrine cysts, papillary apocrine metaplasia, sclerosing adenosis, and duct stasis

Fibroadenomas

KEY FACTS

- Clinical
  - Hard, movable mass in younger patient
  - May present in older women on hormone replacement therapy
  - Hormonally mediated (cyclic) changes in size and associated tenderness
  - Multiplicity (7% to 16%)
  - "Complex" fibroadenomas may have an associated increased breast cancer risk.
  - Giant fibroadenomas: 8 to 10 cm in size

- Mammography
  - Variable appearance
  - Mass or masses: variable size, marginal characteristics and density
  - Mass or masses with punctate (pleomorphic) calcifications
  - Mass or masses with coarse "popcorn" calcification—more common in older women (with hyalinization of fibroadenoma)
  - Punctate (pleomorphic) calcifications without a perceptible mass
  - Coarse "popcorn" calcification in isolation of a mass

- Ultrasound
  - Variable appearance
  - Homogeneously hypoechoic, elliptic mass with no posterior acoustic enhancement or shadowing
  - May have heterogeneous echo texture, some with small cystic components
  - Posterior acoustic enhancement and shadowing may be prominent features.

- Gross
  - Bulging, white, firm tumor

- Histology
  - Lobular derivatives under estrogenic stimulation; hyalinization and regression of epithelial elements after menopause (particularly in women not on estrogen replacement)
  - Proliferation of lobular elements (epithelial and mesenchymal—intralobular stroma) in an expansile fashion
  - Normal two-cell-layer arrangement of epithelial elements (epithelial and myo-epithelial cells)
  - Stromal proliferation around tubular (pericanalicular) or compressed (intracanalicular) ducts
  - Calcification may develop in the stroma (coarse) and within the epithelial elements (punctate, pleomorphic).

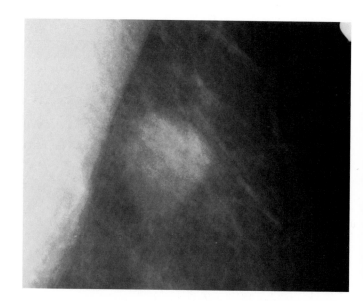

FIGURE 10-11
Fibroadenoma. Well-defined, low-density mass.

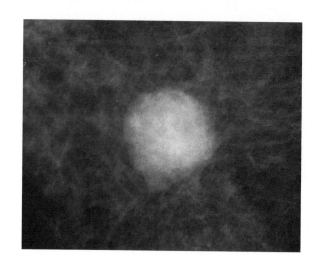

FIGURE 10-12
Fibroadenoma. Well-defined, lobulated mass.

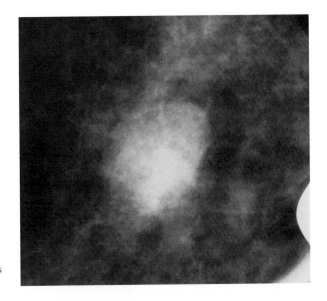

FIGURE 10-13
Fibroadenoma. Mass with partially obscured borders (on spot compression views).

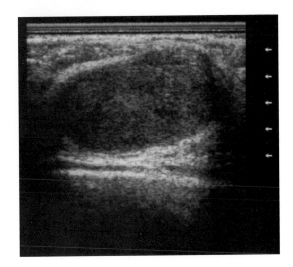

FIGURE 10-14
Fibroadenoma. Well-defined, hypoechoic, oval (wider than tall) mass with posterior acoustic enhancement (variably seen).

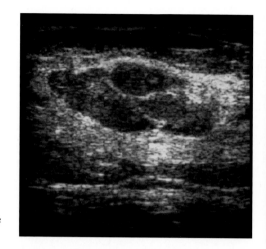

FIGURE 10-15
Fibroadenoma. Well-defined, hypoechoic, oval (wider than tall) mass. Fibrous septations (hyperechoic bands) are
seen in some fibroadenomas.

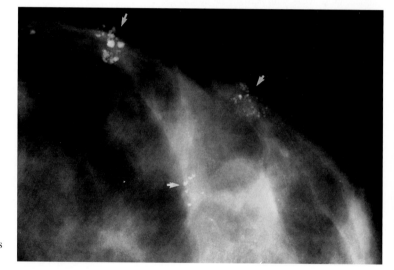

FIGURE 10-16
Fibroadenomas. Multiple fibroadenomas in various stages of hyalinization—calcification (*arrows*). Coarse,
dense calcifications. As in this patient, the calcifications are not always
associated with a soft-tissue mass.

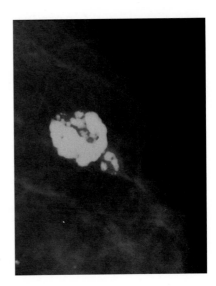

FIGURE 10-17
Fibroadenoma. ''Popcorn''-type calcification. Hyalinized fibroadenoma.

Complex Fibroadenomas

KEY FACTS

- Described and defined by Dupont and colleagues (see Bibliography)
- Fibroadenomas containing:
  - Cysts greater than 3 mm
  - Sclerosing adenosis
  - Epithelial calcifications
  - Papillary apocrine changes
- Parenchyma adjacent to fibroadenomas should be evaluated and characterized as:
  - Free of proliferative changes
  - Proliferative changes with no atypia
  - Proliferative changes with atypia
- Approximately 33% of all fibroadenomas are complex.
- Relative risk of breast cancer
  - 2.17 × in women with noncomplex fibroadenomas
  - 3.10 × in women with complex fibroadenomas
  - 3.72 × in women with complex fibroadenomas and a positive family history
  - 3.88 × in women with complex fibroadenomas and benign proliferative changes in surrounding stroma

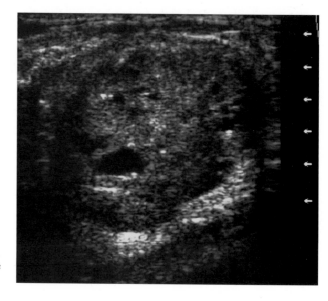

FIGURE 10-18
Fibroadenoma. Round mass with heterogeneous echo texture and cystic component. In most patients, however, we cannot distinguish noncomplex fibroadenomas from complex fibroadenomas. Some posterior acoustic enhancement.

Juvenile Fibroadenoma

KEY FACTS

- Clinical
  - Rapid growth, attaining a massive size with stretching of the overlying skin, dilatation of the superficial veins, and nipple displacement
  - To be distinguished from adolescent breast hypertrophy (bilateral diffuse breast enlargement with no discrete mass, skin stretching, venous distention, or nipple displacement)
- Ultrasound
  - Solid, hypoechoic mass
- Histology
  - Not a specific histologic entity
  - More commonly pericanalicular-type fibroadenoma; dense, cellular stroma
  - Hyperplasia of epithelial elements

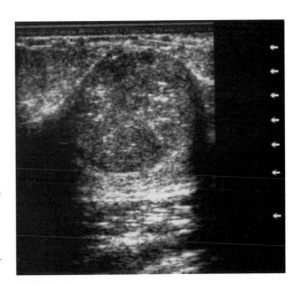

FIGURE 10-19
Fibroadenoma. Palpable, round mass in adolescent woman associated with posterior acoustic enhancement. Fibroadenomas in young women may have a more cellular stroma (phyllodes may be considered). Other than the age of the patient and, at times, a more cellular stroma on histology, these lesions are indistinguishable from fibroadenomas occurring in older women.

Phyllodes Tumor (Cystosarcoma)

KEY FACTS

- Clinical
  - 0.3% of all breast tumors
  - Resembles fibroadenoma
  - Patients typically 15 to 20 years older (mean age: mid-40s) than women with fibroadenomas; malignant variants in slightly older patients
  - Palpable mass (may be large)
  - 3% to 12% of patients have metastasis (hematogeneously)
- Mammography
  - Lesions greater than 3 cm in size more likely to be malignant
  - Circumscribed mass; a few calcify
- Ultrasound
  - Hypoechoic, well-circumscribed mass
  - Lesions with cystic spaces more likely to be malignant
- Gross
  - Tan, gray, or yellow
  - May see cystic and gelatinous portions
  - Leaf-like processes protruding into cystic spaces
- Histology
  - Benign epithelial elements and a cellular stroma; differentiation from fibroadenoma is subjective based on estimates of stromal cellularity and presence of leaf-like processes protruding into cystic spaces
  - Two cell epithelial layers line ducts and cover leaf-like processes.
  - Spindle cells in stroma, atypia, and multinucleated cells can be seen.
  - Lesions are assessed for stromal cellularity, cellular atypia, mitotic rate, and border features of tumor (expansile, infiltrative); size alone is not a criterion for diagnosis.
  - Biologic behavior is difficult to establish. Low-grade lesions are characterized by expansile growth, mild atypia, and less than three mitotic figures per ten high-power fields; these lesions may recur locally and are unlikely to metastasize. High-grade lesions are characterized by an expansile or infiltrative growth pattern, moderate to severe atypia, and three or more mitotic figures per ten high-power fields.

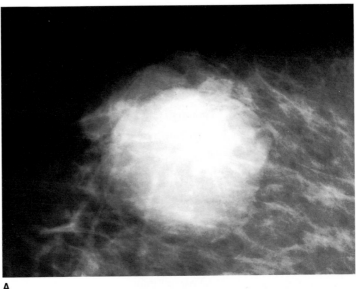

A

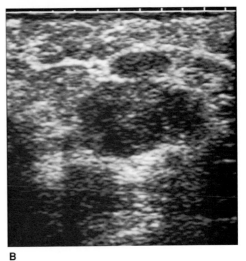

B

FIGURE 10-20
Phyllodes tumor. (**A**) Well-defined mass. (**B**) Well-circumscribed, oval, hypoechoic mass. In some patients, you may see cystic spaces within the mass.

Tubular Adenoma

KEY FACTS

- Clinical
  - Freely movable mass
- Mammography
  - Well-defined mass, may be lobulated
- Ultrasound
  - Oval, hypoechoic mass, homogeneous echo texture
  - Well circumscribed
- Histology
  - Well circumscribed (no true capsule)
  - Densely packed, uniformly small, round, proliferating tubules
  - Two cell linings; no vacuole formation
  - Sparse intervening stroma

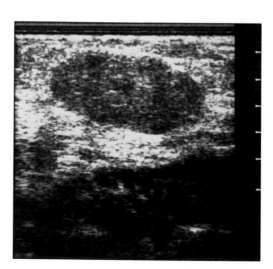

FIGURE 10-21
Tubular adenoma. Well-defined, hypoechoic mass with some posterior acoustic enhancement.

Lactating Adenoma

KEY FACTS

- Clinical
  - Patients are pregnant or nursing.
  - Well-defined, movable mass
  - May enlarge rapidly during pregnancy
  - May be multiple

- Ultrasound
  - Because patients present during or immediately after pregnancy, mammography may not be done.
  - Macrolobulated, oval, well-defined, hypoechoic mass
  - Posterior acoustic enhancement
  - Hyperechoic bands coursing through mass

- Histology
  - Well defined (but no true capsule)
  - Lobulated margin
  - Tubules distended with variable secretory activity (depending on stage of pregnancy or lactation when biopsied)
  - Epithelial lining cells show vacuolization and mitotic activity.
  - May be associated with fibrotic bands (explains hyperechoic bands seen on ultrasound)
  - 5% show areas of infarction.

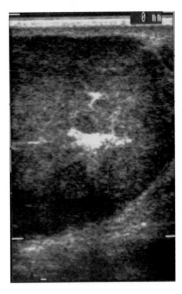

FIGURE 10-22
Lactating adenoma. Large, well-defined mass with posterior acoustic enhancement. Hyperechoic, fibrous bands coursing through lesion.

Sclerosing Adenosis

KEY FACTS

- "Adenosis" refers to proliferation of glandular elements.
- Clinical
    - Most patients asymptomatic (abnormal screening studies)
    - Palpable mass uncommon ("adenosis tumor" described by Haagensen)
    - Controversy as to whether this is an involutional or proliferative process
    - Considered a marker of slightly (1.5 to 2 ×) increased relative risk for subsequent breast cancer
- Mammography
    - Most common pattern: cluster of discrete, punctate, pleomorphic calcifications
    - Smudgy, ill-defined calcifications—wide area of dense breast tissue. This can resemble milk of calcium, but unlike milk of calcium, which has a differential appearance between CC and 90° lateral views, with this type of sclerosing adenosis the calcifications are smudgy on CC, MLO, and 90° lateral views.
    - Mass well defined to spiculated (uncommon presentation)
- Ultrasound
    - Hypoechoic mass
- Histology
    - Proliferation of closely packed lobular units elongated and distorted as a result of compression by surrounding stroma
    - Two cell layers in epithelial elements; may be hyperplasia of myoepithelial cells
    - May be focal or diffuse and florid
    - May extend into perineural spaces (2% of women)

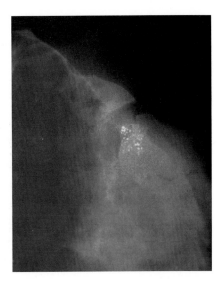

FIGURE 10-23
Sclerosing adenosis. Punctate calcifications in a
tight cluster; even small calcifications have
high density.

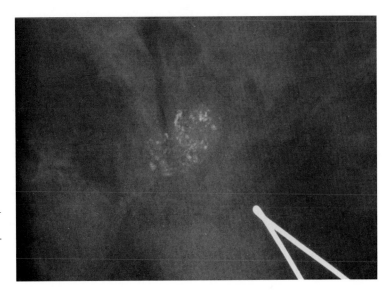

FIGURE 10-24
Sclerosing adenosis. Pleomorphic calcifications. Differential includes hya-
linizing fibroadenoma, papilloma, ductal hyperplasia, fat necrosis, well-
differentiated ductal carcinoma in
situ.

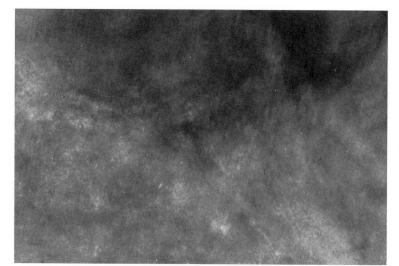

FIGURE 10-25
Sclerosing adenosis. Smudgy calcifications. In contrast to milk of calcium, this appearance in seen in both craniocaudal and 90° lateral views. This process is usually diffuse and bilateral in the setting of dense breast tissue.

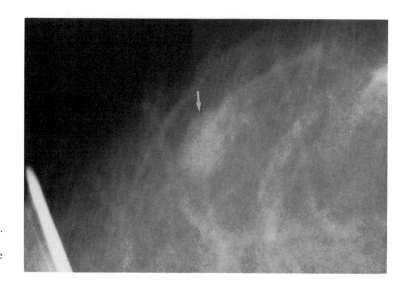

FIGURE 10-26
Sclerosing adenosis. Mass with obscured borders on spot compression. Spiculation sometimes seen. Adenosis tumors are uncommon. In some patients the mass is palpable.

Lobular Neoplasia

KEY FACTS

- Synonymous with lobular carcinoma in situ (LCIS)
- Because this is not a true cancer, "carcinoma" should not be used in describing this entity. As proposed by Haagensen, lobular neoplasia (although not an ideal term either) may be a more appropriate term.
- Often bilateral, multifocal
- Incidental pathologic finding
- More common in premenopausal women; many of these lesions are thought to regress after menopause (unless there is estrogen replacement therapy)
- Biologic behavior different from that of most ductal carcinomas in situ (ductal carcinoma in situ considered a true breast cancer)
- Significant risk marker lesion for subsequent development of breast cancer
- Increased risk applies to both breasts (not limited to breast with diagnosis of lobular neoplasia).
- Cancers that develop may be either ductal or lobular.
- If this is the only diagnosis given in a biopsy done for clinical or mammographic findings, there is no explanation for what prompted the biopsy in the first place. Lobular neoplasia is an incidental histologic diagnosis with no clinical or mammographic findings.
- Lobular neoplasia should not be counted as a positive biopsy in clinical or mammographic series. It is not a cancer, and the abnormality that prompted the biopsy is usually something other than the lobular neoplasia.
- Mammography
  - No abnormality
- Gross
  - No visible lesion
- Histology
  - Uniform cell population distending and distorting at least half the acini in the lobular unit
- Management
  - Controversial
  - Periodic follow-up (clinical, mammographic)
  - Bilateral mastectomy (unilateral mastectomy not appropriate because the increased breast cancer risk applies to both breasts)

Invasive Lobular Carcinoma

KEY FACTS

- Clinical
  - 10% to 15% of all breast cancers; 2% of all breast cancers in women less than age 35; 11% of all breast cancers in women over age 75
  - Bilaterality is high (6% to 28%)
  - Given histologic features, clinical and mammographic diagnosis often difficult
  - Findings can be overlooked because a discrete mass may not be palpated.
  - Areas of thickening or induration are described.
  - Some women present with an area of focal tenderness.
  - Metastatic lobular carcinoma may simulate ovarian cancer—pleural and peritoneal studding with pleural effusions and ascites; involvement of leptomeninges, uterus, and ovaries. In contrast, metastatic disease from invasive ductal carcinoma usually involves solid organs (eg, liver, bone, brain).

- Mammography
  - Spiculated mass (Susan Komen Breast Center [SKBC] 40%)
  - Parenchymal asymmetry (SKBC 16%)
  - Architectural distortion (SKBC 15%)
  - Diffuse breast changes, including decreased breast size and concomitant density increases (SKBC 11%)
  - Relatively well-circumscribed mass (SKBC 11%)
  - Although microcalcifications have been described as a finding for invasive lobular carcinoma, in our experience invasive lobular carcinomas do not develop or present with calcifications. Given the histologic behavior of classic infiltrating lobular carcinoma, the lack of calcification is not surprising.
  - Normal (SKBC 3%)

- Ultrasound
  - Hypoechoic mass may be seen in area of asymmetry, palpable induration, or focal tenderness.
  - Many invasive lobular carcinomas produce striking shadowing.

- Gross
  - Poorly defined area of induration may be apparent; relatively well-circumscribed mass sometimes present

- Histology
  - Small, monomorphic cells infiltrating the stroma in single file
  - Targetoid appearance produced by circumferential infiltration around ducts and lobules by abnormal cells
  - Given small, round monomorphic appearance of the malignant cells, lymphoma is in the differential.
  - Associated lobular neoplasia and atypical lobular hyperplasia may be present.
  - Variants include alveolar, solid, and mixed/atypical.

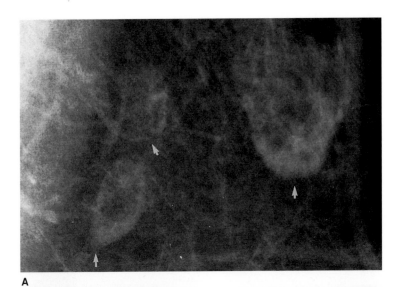

A

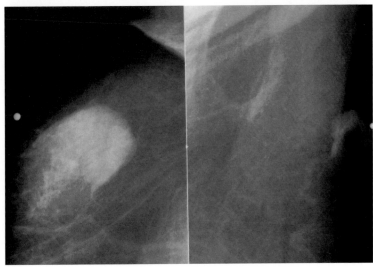

B

FIGURE 11-7
(**A**) Lymph nodes (*arrows*). Masses of mixed density. Size and proportion of soft tissue and fatty hilum vary. (**B**) Enlarging lymph node. Although some fat remains in the hilum, a biopsy was recommended because of size and density increases. Reactive lymph node on histology. Lymph nodes can vary in size between examinations, sometimes going away completely only to reappear on subsequent studies. However, if there is loss of the fatty hilum, rounding, and increasing density, biopsy should be considered.

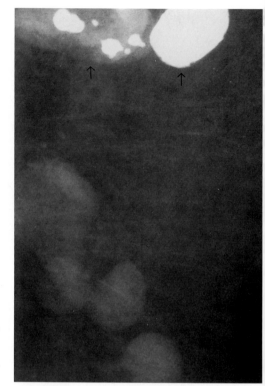

FIGURE 11-8
Calcified lymph nodes (*arrows*).
Coarse calcifications involving lymph
nodes in a woman with a history of
granulomatous disease. Other noncalcified lymph nodes can be seen inferiorly.

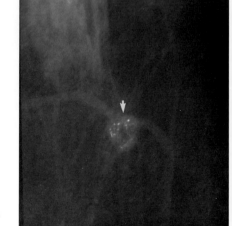

FIGURE 11-9
Gold. Particles of gold in intramammary lymph
node; note central fatty region. This patient with
rheumatoid arthritis was treated with gold. Particles are dense, even the small ones. Usually affects lymph nodes bilaterally. (Courtesy of Dr.
Thomas Getz, Methodist Medical Center, Peoria,
IL)

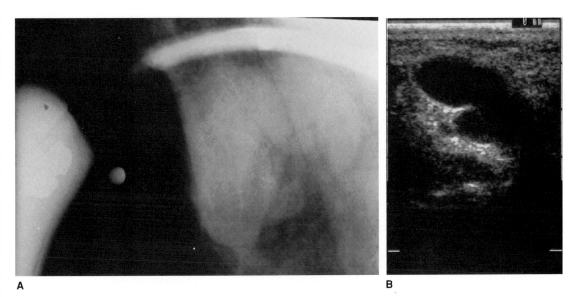

A   B

FIGURE 11-10   Cat scratch disease. (**A**) Spot tangential view of palpable mass (BB). Enlarged, dense, palpable axillary lymph node. No fatty hilum seen. (**B**) Reniform but plump, nearly anechoic mass. Central hyperechoic area still apparent ultrasonographically.

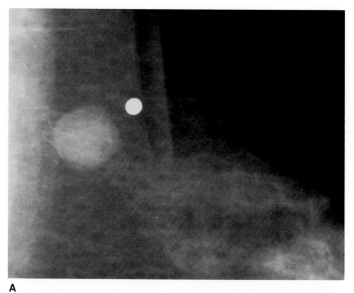

A

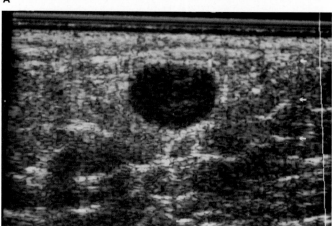

FIGURE 11-11
Reactive lymph node. (**A**) Round, palpable, well-circumscribed mass mammographically (metallic BB marks palpable mass). No fatty hilum identified. (**B**) Round, well-defined, hypoechoic mass. No malignancy histologically.

B

Fat Necrosis

KEY FACTS

- Clinical
  - Nonsuppurative inflammatory process related to trauma or surgery
  - Asymptomatic in most women
  - Palpable mass rarely causes skin retraction when symptomatic.
  - Less commonly associated with ecchymosis, erythema, induration, skin thickening, and adenopathy

- Mammography
  - Spiculated mass with dense center
  - Spiculated mass with variable amounts of central lucency
  - Irregular mass with or without associated calcifications
  - Oil cyst: round, smooth-bordered (thin ''capsule'') lucent mass; calcification of fibrous rim (eggshell or rim calcifications)
  - Cluster of microcalcifications—pleomorphic (indeterminate)
  - Coarse microcalcifications (in some women may develop in oil cysts or masses)
  - After seatbelt injury, a band-like area of increased density occurs. If the patient was the driver, findings are localized to the upper inner or central part of the left breast or the lower inner part of the right breast. If the patient was a front-seat passenger, findings are localized to the upper inner part of the right breast or the lower part of the left breast.

- Ultrasound
  - When the mammographic finding is a spiculated mass, an irregular, hypoechoic mass with a variable amount of shadowing is found on ultrasound.
  - When the mammographic finding is an oil cyst, an anechoic, round, well-defined mass is found on ultrasound, with or without posterior acoustic enhancement or shadowing.
  - Complex mass: internal echoes or intracystic soft-tissue component

- Histology
  - Fat cell death with vacuole formation
  - Fibroblasts, lipid-laden macrophages, and multinucleated giant cells surround dying fat cells.
  - Fibrosis
  - Calcifications may develop, initially pleomorphic. With regression they may solidify, the end point being coarse dystrophic calcifications.

(text continues on the next page)

Fat Necrosis *(Continued)*

- Oil cysts
  - Liquefaction of fatty tissue (contents: triglycerides)
  - It is unclear if these all arise from fat necrosis. Given their presence in patients with steatocystoma multiplex, some may arise independent of trauma or surgery.
  - May be palpable
  - Lucent tissue with thin fibrous "capsule" seen mammographically
  - Nearly anechoic mass on ultrasound; some are anechoic with hyperechoic intracystic soft-tissue component
  - Thick, oily material obtained on aspiration

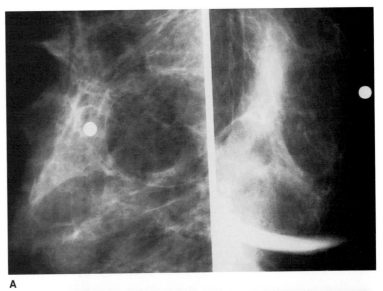

A

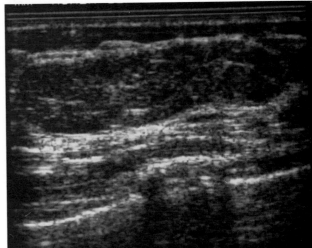

FIGURE 11-14
Lipoma. (**A**) Right mediolateral oblique view back to back with right craniocaudal view. Palpable (metallic BB), well-defined, lucent mass. Fatty tissue delineated by a thin fibrous band. (**B**) Oval hypoechoic mass corresponding to the palpable area. Unlike oil cysts, which simulate cysts on ultrasound, lipomas are solid, hypoechoic or hyperechoic masses on ultrasound.

B

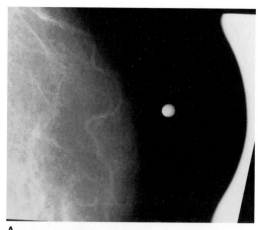

A

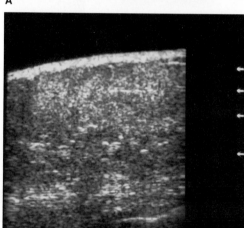

FIGURE 11-15
Lipoma. (**A**) Left craniocaudal spot, tangential view (BB marks palpable area). Only fatty tissue is imaged. (**B**) Oval hyperechoic mass corresponding to palpable mass.

B

Hamartoma (Fibroadenolipoma)

KEY FACTS

- Clinical
  - "Breast within a breast"
  - Palpable mass

- Mammography
  - Seemingly encapsulated glandular and fatty tissue
  - Breast cancer can arise in the glandular elements of a hamartoma.

- Ultrasound
  - Normal breast tissue, no distinctive features

- Histology
  - Variable, partial or complete encapsulation of normal breast tissue. Fibrocystic changes, including cyst formation and sclerosing adenosis, may be seen within the nodule.
  - Overgrowth of mature breast cells and tissue; one element may predominate

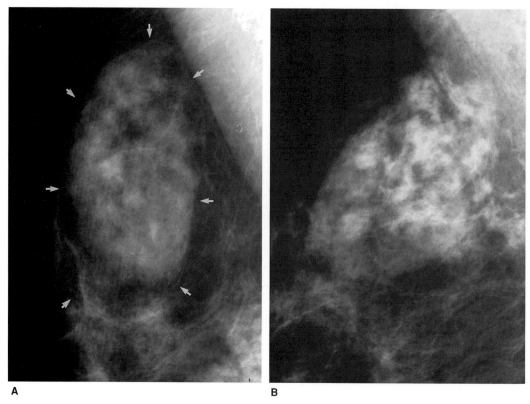

A   **B**

FIGURE 11-16   Hamartoma (fibroadenolipoma). (**A**) Right exaggerated craniocaudal view. Glandular and fatty elements (*arrows*) in upper lateral portion of right breast (''breast within a breast''). These are sometimes palpable. (**B**) Right mediolateral oblique view. Glandular and fatty elements in upper lateral portion of right breast (''breast within a breast'').

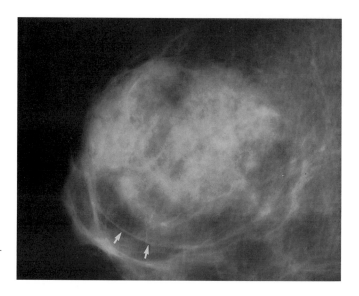

FIGURE 11-17
Hamartoma (fibroadenolipoma). Seemingly encapsulated (*arrows*) glandular and fatty tissue (mixed density).

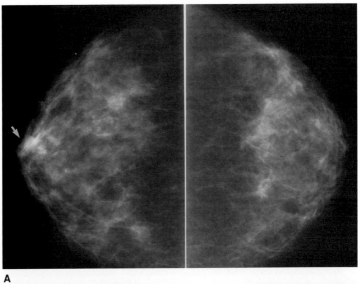

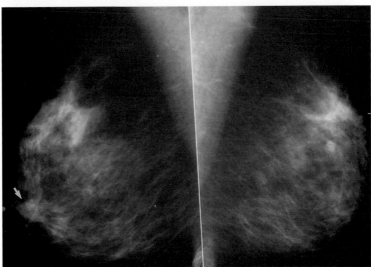

FIGURE 11-20
Abscess. (**A**) Right and left cranio-caudal views. Palpable mass (*arrow*) in right subareolar area. (**B**) Right and left mediolateral oblique views. Palpable mass (metallic BB) in right subareolar area (*arrow*).

(continued)

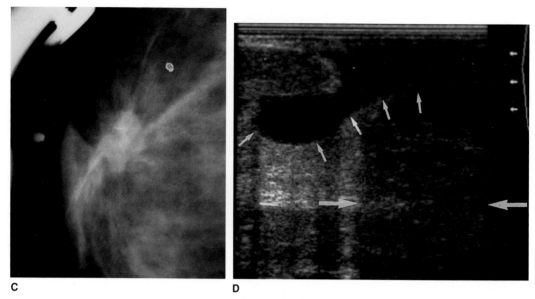

FIGURE 11-20   **(CONTINUED)** **(C)** Right subareolar spot compression view. Spiculated mass confirmed on spot compression views. Nipple skin thickening. **(D)** Nearly anechoic mass with duct extending to nipple (*small arrows*). Note shadowing produced by nipple (*bracketed by large white arrows*).

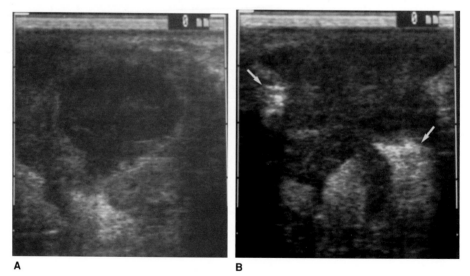

FIGURE 11-21   Abscess. **(A)** Irregular mass with thickened wall and central fluid collection. **(B)** Irregular, heterogeneous mass with thickened wall and central fluid collection. Hyperechoic bands (*arrows*) some with shadowing consistent with air.

Pseudoangiomatous Stromal Hyperplasia

KEY FACTS

- Clinical
  - More common in premenopausal women
  - Palpable mass
  - May recur locally (15% to 22%)
  - Hormonal etiology; possibly a response to progesterone in estrogen-stimulated tissue
  - Multifocal in up to 60% of women
  - Not considered premalignant or associated with malignancy

- Mammography
  - Well- or partially circumscribed mass

- Ultrasound
  - Solid, well-defined, hypoechoic mass (may have heterogeneous echo pattern)

- Histology
  - Variable size, from microscopic to several centimeters; microscopic lesions common
  - Must be distinguished from low-grade angiosarcoma
  - A complex pattern of anastomosing channels is formed by the disruption and separation of collagen fibers in the interlobular and intralobular stroma.
  - Spaces are lined incompletely by spindled myofibroblasts simulating endothelial cells (pseudovascular) and contain mucopolysaccharides. A similar pattern is seen during the luteal phase of the menstrual cycle.
  - Immunohistologic staining for endothelial markers (eg, factor VIII) is negative in these lesions.

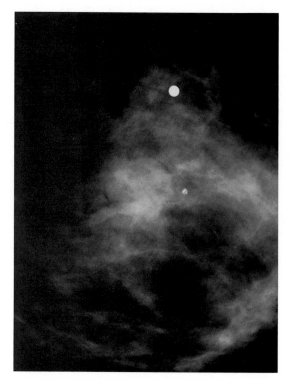

FIGURE 11-22
Pseudoangiomatous stromal hyperplasia. Partially defined (halo)
mass. Some of the border is obscured.

Suture Calcifications

KEY FACTS

- Clinical
    - These are more common after lumpectomy and radiation therapy; radiation damage to tissue delays the resorption of suture material, permitting calcium deposition. They can, however, be seen after biopsy (with benign histology).
    - Catgut sutures have been proposed as a nidus for calcium precipitation.

- Mammography
    - Curvilinear calcifications forming loops
    - Coarse linear calcifications (nonanatomic distribution), smooth border limited to area of surgery
    - Calcified knots; may be evenly spaced

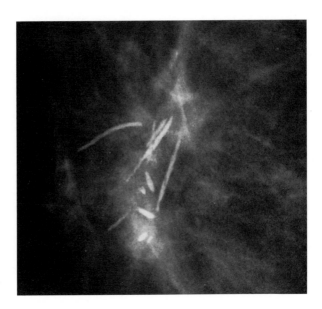

FIGURE 11-23
Suture calcifications. Coarse, linear calcifications, smooth border. Nonanatomic distribution in area of previous surgery. In some women, knots can be seen in suture.

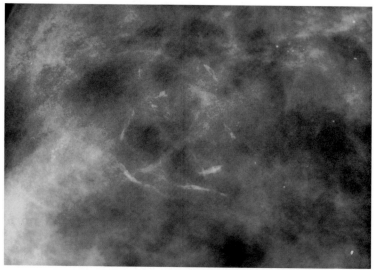

A

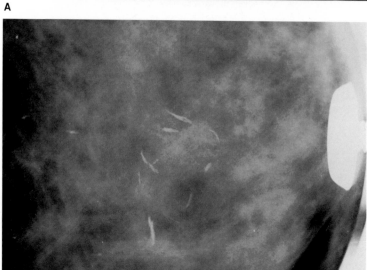

FIGURE 11-24

Suture calcifications. (**A**) Developing linear calcifications at previous biopsy site. (**B**) One year after **A** (2 years after benign biopsy), calcification is continuing. Coarse, linear calcifications with smooth border.

B

Hemangioma

KEY FACTS

- Clinical
  - Variable incidence (1.2% to 11%)
  - Some are incidental histologic findings; others present with a palpable mass.

- Mammography
  - Normal
  - Well-circumscribed, macrolobulated mass; may have associated punctate calcifications
  - Punctate microcalcifications in isolation of a mass

- Histology
  - Perilobular: small (0.5 to 4.0 mm), easily overlooked; ill-defined margins; endothelial cells, no atypia
  - Cavernous, capillary, juvenile, and venous: greater than 5 mm in size; well-defined margins; cavernous have dilated vessels, normal endothelial cells; capillary have capillary-sized vessels, normal endothelial cells; juvenile have immature capillary hemangioma; venous have thick-walled vessels (elastic vessel wall)
  - Less than a low-power microscopic field in diameter
  - Well circumscribed, perilobular
  - Uniform vascular spaces
  - No atypical endothelial cells
  - Scant connective tissue stroma
  - Multiple lesions
  - Bilateral in some women

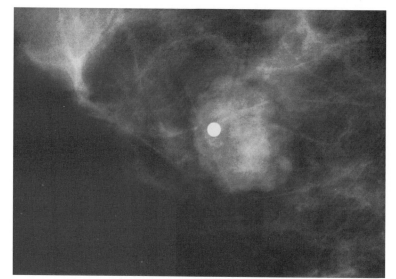

FIGURE 11-25
Cavernous hemangioma. Metallic BB marks palpable mass. Well-defined, lobulated mass mammographically. These lesions are not typically palpable. Histologically, small (mammographically occult) lesions are common.

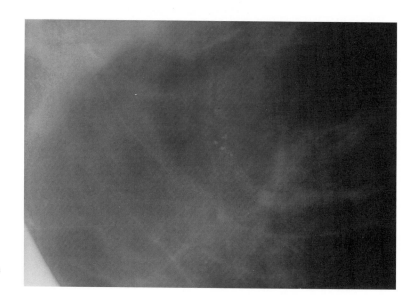

FIGURE 11-26
Capillary hemangioma. Punctate cluster of microcalcifications.

Diabetic Fibrous Breast Disease

KEY FACTS

- Clinical
  - Early onset, longstanding insulin-dependent diabetes mellitus
  - Hard, ill-defined, nontender mass, uni- or bilateral
  - No data on incidence but may be more common than thought

- Mammography
  - Dense breast tissue
  - Vascular calcifications (diabetic patients)

- Ultrasound
  - Significant shadowing in area of clinical concern

- Histology
  - Dense stromal fibrosis
  - Ductal and lobular obliteration
  - Perivascular and periductal lymphocytic infiltration
  - Possible autoimmune disorder

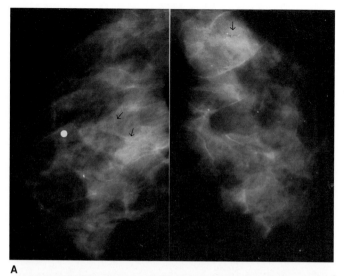

A

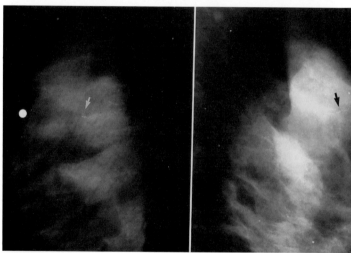

B

FIGURE 11-27

Diabetic fibrous mastopathy. (**A**)
Right and left craniocaudal views
back to back. Metallic BB marks
palpable mass. Dense tissue with
no discrete abnormality mammographically. Arrows mark vascular
(quirky) calcifications in a 40-year-
old. The tip-off is the patient's
young age. In a young patient, vascular calcifications may be related
to an underlying metabolic disorder
(in this patient, insulin-dependent diabetes). (**B**) Right and left mediolateral oblique views back to back.
Metallic BB marks palpable mass.
Dense tissue with no discrete abnormality mammographically. Arrows
mark vascular (quirky) calcifications. (**C**) Acoustic shadowing
when palpable mass is scanned.

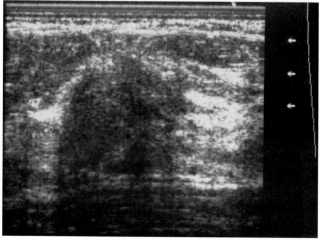

C

Extraabdominal Desmoid

KEY FACTS

- Clinical
  - Fibromatosis
  - Associated with Gardner's syndrome
  - Locally aggressive; requires wide excision
  - May recur (20%), usually within first 5 years
  - May be related to previous trauma or surgery; have been reported in women with saline implants
- Mammography
  - Spiculated mass
- Ultrasound
  - Hypoechoic mass with variable acoustic shadowing
- Histology
  - Ill defined; variable cellularity
  - Proliferation of fibroblasts (admixture of fibroblasts and myofibroblasts)

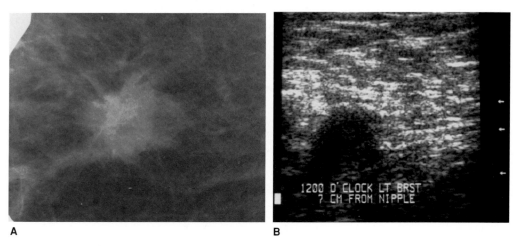

A   B

FIGURE 11-28   Extraabdominal desmoid. (**A**) Spiculated mass. These commonly arise close to the pectoral muscle. (**B**) Hypoechoic mass with posterior acoustic shadowing.

Lymphoma

KEY FACTS

- Clinical
  - Primary in breast, if widespread or prior extramammary lymphoma excluded
  - Primary breast lymphoma rare (0.1% to 0.5%); secondary involvement more common
  - Primary breast lymphoma accounts for 2.5% of all extranodal forms of lymphoma.
  - 30% to 40% axillary involvement
  - 13% bilaterality
  - 10% present with night sweats, fever, and weight loss.
  - Although experience is limited, estrogen- and progesterone-receptor positivity has been reported.
  - Two divergent clinical patterns: diffuse large cell of B-cell origin (commonly unilateral, broad age spectrum, variable course); Burkitt's type (rapidly fatal course, develops bilaterally in pregnant or lactating women, ovarian and CNS involvement)

- Mammography
  - Mass or multiple masses, well circumscribed to spiculated, variable size
  - Diffuse increase in parenchymal density
  - Skin thickening

- Ultrasound
  - Well-defined to irregular hypoechoic mass or masses

- Histology
  - May be difficult to differentiate from medullary carcinoma, but epithelial markers absent in lymphomas

- Pseudolymphoma (lymphoid pseudotumor)
  - Large mass (2.5 to 5 cm), rapid development
  - May represent an overwhelming response to trauma; also associated with anti-convulsive therapy
  - Irregular mass mammographically (nonspecific)
  - Ultrasonographically, echogenic (isoechoic with glandular tissue, hyperechoic relative to subcutaneous fat) tissue with hypoechoic, ''reticular'' bands representing lymphocytic infiltrate
  - Aggregation of nonneoplastic lymphocytes (more commonly involving GI tract [stomach] and lung)

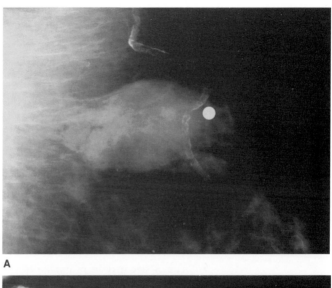

A

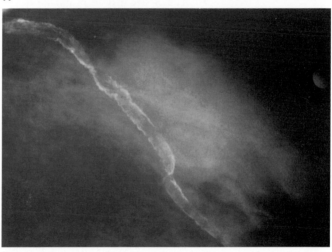

B

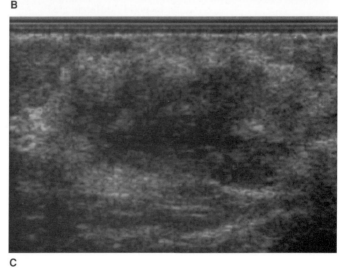

C

FIGURE 11-29
Lymphoma. (**A**) Metallic BB marks palpable area. Partially defined mass on routine view. (**B**) Spot magnification view. Indistinct margins. (**C**) Irregular hypoechoic mass.

Angiosarcoma

KEY FACTS

- Less than 0.05% of all primary breast cancers
- Clinical
  - Younger women (average age 35)
  - Painless, discrete mass
  - Diffuse breast enlargement (approximately 12%)
  - In superficial lesions, a bluish-red discoloration of overlying skin may be present.
  - Vascular metastasis, bypass axillary lymph nodes (axillary dissection therefore not done)
  - Contralateral breast involvement reportedly common
  - Tumor size may be of prognostic significance.
- Mammography
  - Microlobulated, irregular mass (''cloud-like'') may have associated coarse calcifications.
- Gross
  - Poorly defined mass
  - Soft, spongy consistency with hemorrhagic areas
- Histology
  - Irregular, anastomosing vascular channels lined by hyperchromatic, atypical endothelial cells permeating breast parenchyma
  - Solid nests of spindle cells
  - Based on amount of solid, spindle-cell component and tufting of atypical endothelial cells, angiosarcomas can be divided in type I, II, or III (well-, moderately, or poorly differentiated).
- Angiosarcoma associated with lymphedema (Stewart-Treves)
  - Develops in women with chronic lymphedema most commonly (90%) after radical mastectomy and axillary nodal dissection with or without radiation therapy for breast cancer
  - Also reported in patients with lymphedema from other causes (eg, after treatment for melanoma or congenital lymphedema)
  - Develops 10 to 20 years or more after treatment
  - Initial focal purple discoloration progresses into plaques and nodules, with ulceration and bleeding.

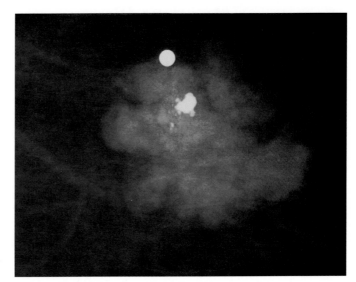

FIGURE 11-30
Angiosarcoma. Metallic BB marks palpable area. Macrolobulated, well-defined mass (''cloud-like'')—common appearance for vascular lesions—with coarse calcifications. Skin coloration (bluish) may be clinically apparent in area of palpable mass.

Metastatic Disease

KEY FACTS

- Clinical
  - The most common metastatic lesion is metastatic cancer from the contralateral breast, through lymphatic channels of the anterior chest.
  - Extramammary metastases uncommon (1.2% of cancers in the breast); hematogenous
  - Hematopoietic and lymphoreticular
  - Melanoma
  - Lung
  - Ovarian, stomach, cervical
  - Palpable mass
- Mammography
  - Round, well- to ill-defined mass—commonly, multiple small bilateral masses
- Ultrasound
  - Solid, hypoechoic mass
- Histology
  - Well demarcated, lacking an intraductal or lobular component

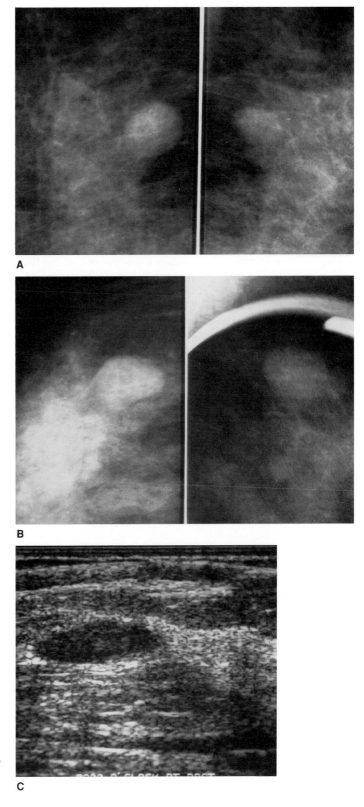

FIGURE 11-31
Metastatic melanoma. (**A**) Right craniocaudal (CC) views 1 year apart back to
back. Mass increasing in size. (**B**) Routine right CC and spot compression
view back to back. Margins of mass partially obscured. (**C**) Oval, hypoechoic
mass.

BIBLIOGRAPHY

Adler DD. Mammographic evaluation of masses. RSNA Categorical Course in Breast Imaging Syllabus 1995, pp 107–116

Bohman LG, Bassett LW, Gold RH, Volt R. Breast metastases from extramammary malignancies. Radiology 1982;144:309–312

Cardenosa G, Eklund GW. Breast anatomy, histology and cancer. RSNA Categorical Course in Breast Imaging Syllabus 1995, pp 21–28

Cardenosa G, Eklund GW. Imaging the altered breast. In Taveras JM, Ferrucci JT (eds). Radiology: diagnosis, imaging, intervention. Philadelphia, JB Lippincott 1993.

Cohen MA, Morris EA, Rosen PP, Dershaw DD, Liberman L, Abramson AF. Pseudoangiomatous stromal hyperplasia: mammographic, sonographic and clinical patterns. Radiology 1996;198:117–120

Donegan WL. Evaluation of a palpable mass. N Engl J Med 1992;327:937–942

Feig SA. Breast masses: mammographic and sonographic evaluation. Radiol Clin North Am 1992;30:67–92

Helvie MA, Adler DD, Rebner M, Oberman HA. Breast hamartomas: variable mammographic appearance. Radiology 1989;170:417–421

Hogge JP, Robinson RE, Magnant CM, Zuurbier RA. The mammographic spectrum of fat necrosis of the breast. RadioGraphics 1995;15:1347–1356

Liberman LL, Dershaw DD, Kaufman RJ, Rosen PP. Angiosarcoma of the breast. Radiology 1992;183:649–654

Mendelson EB, Doshi N, Grabb BC, Goldfarb WI. Pseudolymphoma of the breast: imaging findings. AJR 1994;162:617–619

Meyer JE, Ferraro FA, Frenna TH, DiPiro PJ, Denison DM. Mammographic appearance of normal intramammary lymph nodes in an atypical location. AJR 1993;161:779–780

Polger MR, Denison CM, Lester S, Meyer JE. Pseudoangiomatous stromal hyperplasia: mammographic and sonographic appearances. AJR 1996;166:349–352

Sickles EA. Breast masses: mammographic evaluation. Radiology 1989;173:297–303

Stacey-Clear A, McCarthy KA, Hall DA, et al. Calcified suture material in the breast after radiation therapy. Radiology 1992;183:207–208

Westinghouse-Logan W, Yanes-Hoffman N. Diabetic fibrous breast disease. Radiology 1989;172:667–670

Breast Imaging Companion
by Gilda Cardenosa
Lippincott-Raven Publishers, Philadelphia © 1997

Chapter 12

THE ALTERED BREAST

General Comments

KEY FACTS

- Surgical procedures or trauma may alter the mammographic appearance of breast tissue. Recognizing these changes is important in avoiding unnecessary evaluation or additional procedures.

- The patient's history and relevant clinical information are often important in evaluating a woman with a history of prior surgery or trauma.

- Knowing histology results from a prior biopsy can be useful in establishing appropriate follow-up or the need for repeat biopsy in some women.

Breast Biopsies

KEY FACTS

- The amount of tissue removed for clinically occult lesions is largely determined by the level of suspicion and the surgical technique.
  - High likelihood of benignity: the lesion and little surrounding tissue should be removed
  - High likelihood of malignancy: the lesion with wide margins should be removed
  - The amount of tissue removed may affect the postoperative changes seen mammographically.

- Mammography
  - No discernible change in more than 50% of women, particularly after accurate localization and minimal-volume biopsies
  - Skin changes: thickening and deformity
  - Parenchymal asymmetry: removal of breast tissue may lead to asymmetries compared with contralateral breast
  - Parenchymal distortion may be associated with skin thickening and dimpling.
  - A spiculated mass (fat necrosis) may be seen in the first year after biopsy. It usually resolves with increasing amounts of fat accumulating in the center of the spiculated area.
  - Dystrophic calcifications may be pleomorphic initially, but with time they coarsen.

- If the biopsy results include nonproliferative benign changes (eg, apocrine metaplasia, sclerosing adenosis, epithelial hyperplasia with no atypia, cysts, fibrosis), the woman is returned to annual screening.

- If a marker lesion (eg, atypical ductal hyperplasia, lobular neoplasia [lobular carcinoma in situ]; we also consider multiple papillomas, radial scar, and complex sclerosing lesions in this category, but not everyone would agree because there are no epidemiologic data supporting this) is diagnosed on histology or if the woman has a significant family history of breast cancer:
  - Follow-up 6 months after biopsy recommended to establish a new baseline for the patient
  - If there is an area of fat necrosis, its appearance is documented early.
  - Confusion in the future (18 to 24 months after biopsy) relative to a spiculated mass at the surgical site can be avoided if 6-month postbiopsy images are available for comparison.
  - Fat necrosis should remain stable or decrease in size and density with time.
  - Rebiopsy should be considered with increasing distortion or density at the biopsy site.

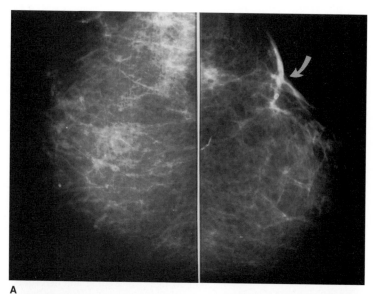

A

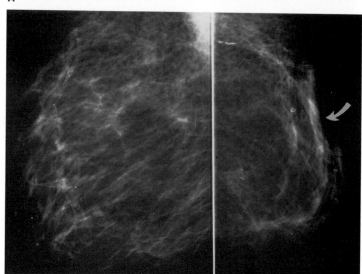

B

FIGURE 12-1
Postbiopsy changes. (**A**) Right and left craniocaudal views. Left breast smaller than right secondary to tissue removal. Skin thickening and deformity at biopsy site (*arrow*). Single round, lucent-centered calcification. (**B**) Right and left mediolateral oblique views. Left breast smaller than right secondary to tissue removal. Skin thickening and deformity at biopsy site (*arrow*). Single round, lucent-centered calcification.

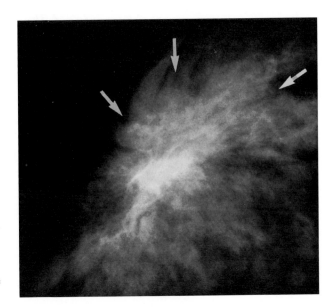

FIGURE 12-2
Postbiopsy changes. Although more than 50% of patients have no appreciable change in the appearance of breast tissue on mammograms after surgery, in some women spiculated masses (simulating malignancy) can be seen at the operative site (*arrows*). Postbiopsy changes should remain stable or decrease in size and density with time.

Lumpectomy and Radiation Therapy

KEY FACTS

GENERAL COMMENTS

- Clinical

    - Conservative breast cancer treatment: excising breast cancer with a wide, tumor-free margin, followed, in most women, by radiation therapy (XRT)

    - Tumor and breast size must be considered so that complete excision can be accomplished with good cosmetic results.

    - Subareolar lesions may require removal of the nipple–areolar complex. Obtaining acceptable cosmetic results may be difficult; nipple reconstruction may be undertaken.

    - Positive axillary lymph nodes are not a contraindication.

    - XRT started 2 to 5 weeks after lumpectomy; 40 to 50 Gy; electron beam boost may bring total to 60 to 66 Gy; axilla not usually radiated

    - Results from seven randomized controlled trials throughout the world have shown no survival difference between mastectomy and conservative treatment (with XRT) in women with tumors less than 5 cm in diameter and no distant disease

    - Mastectomy is usually recommended if a local recurrence develops in a woman after lumpectomy and XRT. The overall survival, even in women with local recurrences, is not significantly different from that of women who have a mastectomy after the initial diagnosis.

- Contraindications (relative)

    - Multicentric (particularly if in different quadrants) or diffuse breast cancer

    - Diagnosis during first or second trimester of pregnancy; if diagnosed during third trimester, XRT can be done after delivery

    - Prior XRT to chest wall (eg, Hodgkin's): adding radiation for breast cancer treatment may result in an unacceptable cumulative dose

    - Collagen vascular disorders

- Local recurrences

    - Recurrence rates are 5% to 10% within 5 years and 10% to 15% at 10 years.

    - The tumor recurs at or close to the lumpectomy site during the first 7 years of follow-up (mean time to recurrence 3 years); after 7 years, tumor recurrence occurs in any quadrant.

    - Increased likelihood of recurrence in women with an invasive cancer having an extensive intraductal component (particularly in young women), large ductal carcinoma in situ (DCIS), inadequate treatment of original tumor (residual disease in breast)

- Mammography

    - Preoperatively: must assess extent of tumor (possibility of extensive intraductal component), possibility of multicentricity, and contralateral breast

    - Accurate preoperative wire localization to ensure complete removal of lesion

- Specimen radiography—although this is a two-dimensional depiction of a three-dimensional structure, evaluate proximity of lesion to margins
- Consider obtaining a mammogram if residual disease is thought to be present in the breast.
- Consider mammogram before starting XRT to document presence of residual calcifications (in women with DCIS).
- If residual calcifications (DCIS) are present, re-excision may be undertaken.

MAMMOGRAPHIC FINDINGS AFTER LUMPECTOMY AND XRT

- Fluid collections
  - Oval mass, dense, well marginated, variable in size (surgical bed allowed to fill in gradually; drains should not be left in place routinely); variable density (within an individual seroma or hematoma and between different fluid collections)
  - Ultrasound: complex cystic mass or masses at lumpectomy site; septations, loculation, thickened wall may be present

- Scar
  - Fluid collections replaced by architectural distortion or spiculated mass (6 to 18 months)
  - Fat trapped in center of mass
  - Change of appearance between views
  - Contract and shrink over time with increasing amounts of fat accumulating in center of scar
  - Consider recurrence with increases in size or density of scar after two stable examinations.

- Edema
  - Breast enlarges; compression may be limited, so adequate exposure may be difficult to obtain.
  - Changes may be more prominent in periareolar and inferior portions of breast.
  - Density increases.
  - Increased density and thickening of trabecula
  - Changes usually resolve within 2 years.

- Skin thickening
  - Follows time course of breast edema
  - Approximately 20% of women have residual skin thickening two years after XRT.
  - Tangential views may be needed if skin changes are superimposed on the lumpectomy site, simulating distortion.
  - Skin thickening is a factor in the overall increased density of the breast after XRT.

(text continues on next page)

Lumpectomy and Radiation Therapy *(Continued)*

- Calcification
  - Magnification views should be done after surgery and before XRT: residual calcifications?
  - Re-excision may be undertaken if residual calcifications (DCIS) are found before XRT.
  - Calcifications related to fat necrosis may be punctate, pleomorphic initially.
  - Dystrophic—round, smooth, some with lucent centers, large, coarse, linear with smooth borders
  - Suture
  - Tumor recurrence—magnification views needed for full evaluation

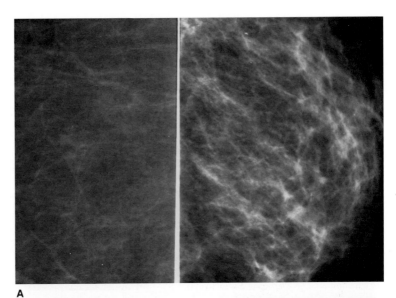

A

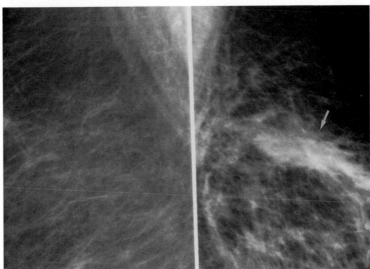

B

FIGURE 12-3
(**A**) Post-radiation therapy (XRT) changes. Right and left craniocaudal views. Trabecular thickening and increased density of left breast compared with right on first examination after completion of XRT. Many of these changes resolve on follow-up studies. (**B**) Postlumpectomy and XRT changes. Right and left mediolateral oblique views. Lumpectomy change (*arrow*). Trabecular thickening and increased density of left breast compared with right on first examination after completion of XRT. Most of these changes resolve on follow-up studies.

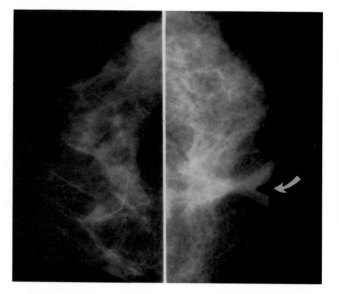

FIGURE 12-4
Postlumpectomy and radiation therapy changes. Right and left craniocaudal views 1 year after surgery. Left breast smaller than right. Architectural distortion, skin thickening, and retraction at lumpectomy site (*arrow*). Diffuse density increase of left breast reflects trabecular thickening and residual skin thickening (two layers of thickened skin are superimposed on the breast parenchyma).

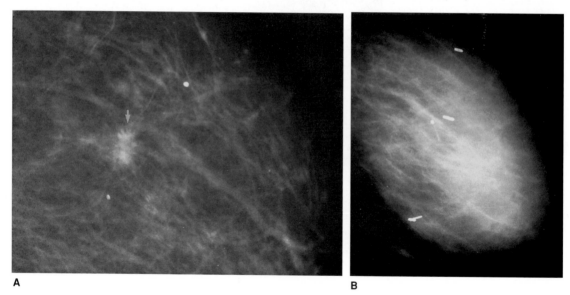

A   B

FIGURE 12-5   (**A**) Infiltrating ductal carcinoma. Spiculated mass detected on screening mammogram (*arrow*). (**B**) Postoperative seroma. Oval, well-circumscribed mass, variable in density; surgical clips at lumpectomy site.

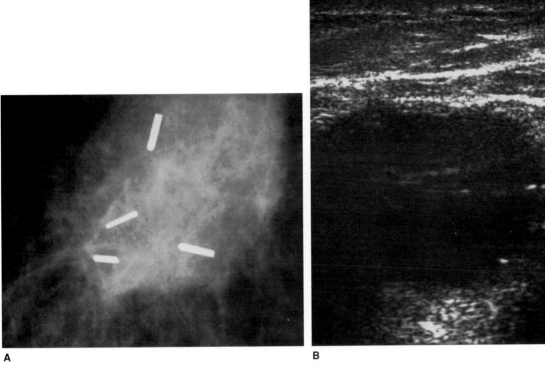

FIGURE 12-6 Postoperative seroma. (**A**) Oval, partially obscured mass, variable in density; surgical clips at lumpectomy site. (**B**) Complex cystic mass on ultrasound.

Mastectomy-Side Views

KEY FACTS

- Clinical

    - A good clinical examination of the mastectomy site will usually detect local recurrences.

    - Without the breast, it is easier to interpose residual fatty tissue between the examining fingers and the chest wall and to palpate any developing mass.

    - A thorough examination is needed, however; otherwise, even clinically apparent lesions may go undetected.

- Mammography

    - Mediolateral oblique (MLO) view of the mastectomy side is advocated by some to detect clinically occult local recurrences.

    - However, several investigators have suggested that this is not cost-effective, as a thorough physical examination will usually identify local recurrences. Others state that in some women, imaging the mastectomy side detects early local recurrences and therefore should be done.

    - Many facilities in the United States do not do images of the mastectomy side.

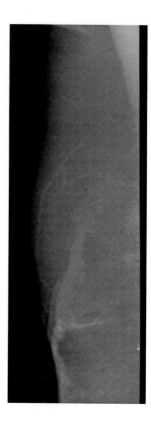

FIGURE 12-7
Mastectomy side. Single mediolateral view. Because in most patients there is only a small amount of fatty tissue on the mastectomy side, even small masses should be readily apparent during a thorough physical examination. Some, however, advocate that these views should be done because early local, clinically occult recurrences may be detected in some patients.

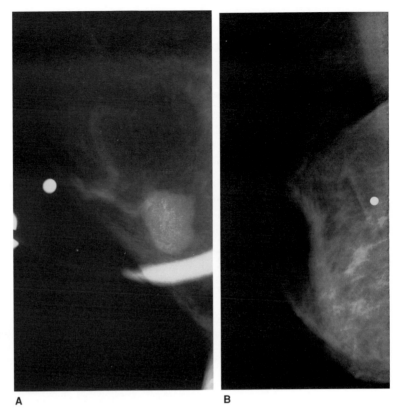

FIGURE 12-8
(**A**) Local recurrence (mucinous carcinoma) on mastectomy side. In this patient, the local recurrence is palpable. Well-circumscribed mass with punctate calcifications. (**B**) Local recurrence (poorly differentiated infiltrating ductal carcinoma). Diffuse trabecular and skin thickening. Clinically apparent.

A

B

Breast Reconstruction

KEY FACTS

* Clinical

    * Some women elect to have reconstruction after mastectomy.

    * Saline and silicone implants (although the FDA has banned the use of silicone implants for esthetic purposes pending further testing, silicone implants may still be used for breast reconstruction after mastectomy) or autologous transplantation (rectus abdominis muscle, latissimus dorsi flap)

    * Expanders are used in some women to expand the skin and chest wall space to accommodate the final implant. Saline can be infused in the expander (through a skin port) over time, thereby gradually expanding the space for the final implant.

    * Depending on breast size, and for symmetry, the contralateral breast may need to be augmented or reduced.

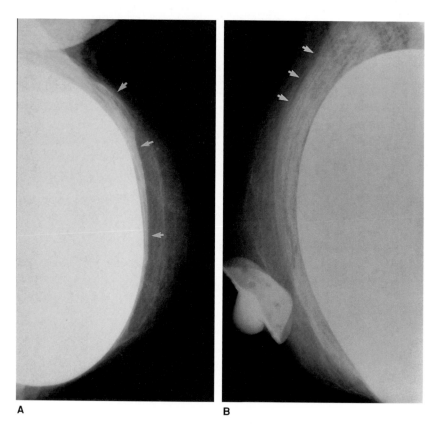

A   B

FIGURE 12-9   Reconstruction. (**A**) Subpectoral silicone implant. Pectoral muscle (*arrows*) coursing anterior to implant. (**B**) Breast and nipple reconstruction after mastectomy. As in most patients with reconstruction, the implant is subpectoral in position. Pectoral muscle coursing over implant (*arrow*).

- Mammography
  - Augmentation implant for reconstruction purposes is usually placed in a subpectoral location.
  - Variable amounts of fat, a soft-tissue density close to the chest wall, and surgical clips are characteristic findings in women who have had autologous transplants (rectus abdominis, latissimus dorsi)
  - There are no data for or against imaging the reconstruction side. The imaging protocol varies by institution, but most do not image the reconstruction side.

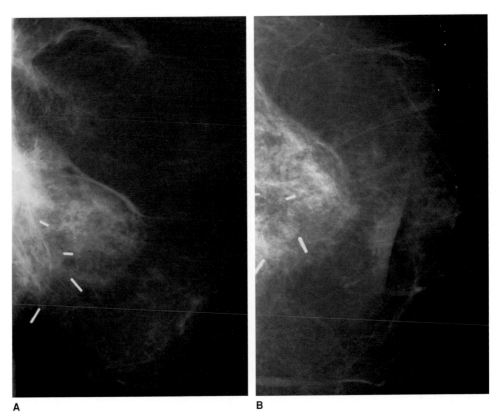

A   B

FIGURE 12-10   Transverse rectus abdominis muscle flap. (**A**) Mediolateral oblique view. Predominantly fatty tissue. Rectus muscle seen as soft-tissue mass-like area close to chest wall. (**B**) Craniocaudal view. Predominantly fatty tissue. Rectus muscle seen as soft-tissue mass-like area close to chest wall. Imaging the reconstruction site may be more appropriate in women with autologous transplants because of the increased tissue overlying chest wall.

Augmentation

KEY FACTS

- Clinical
  - Over 2 million women in the United States have augmentation implants (esthetic).

- Methods
  - Subcutaneous silicone or paraffin injections—not approved in the United States, but still done in some countries
  - Autologous tissue transplants—not generally used for esthetic augmentation; done in some women after mastectomy
  - Implants—silicone, not currently approved by FDA for esthetic augmentation but can be used for reconstruction after mastectomy; or saline implants used

- Implant types
  - Silicone
    - Smooth
    - Polyurethane-coated
    - Textured
    - Double lumen
  - Saline

- Implant placement
  - Subglandular (prepectoral), between glandular tissue and pectoralis major muscle
  - Subpectoral, between pectoralis major and minor muscles

- Implant placement methods
  - Inframammary fold incision
  - Periareolar incision
  - Transaxillary

- Imaging
  - Four views of each breast: two (craniocaudal [CC] and mediolateral oblique [MLO]) with the implant in the field of view and two (CC and MLO) with the implant displaced
  - Additional views undertaken if indicated (eg, spot compression, magnification, tangential)
  - Implant bulging (part of implant protrudes through capsule)
  - Implant wrinkles are seen commonly with saline implants; they occur just as commonly with silicone implants but are not readily apparent on mammograms because of silicone density.
  - Coarse calcification of capsule
  - With rupture, may see extracapsular silicone surrounding implant and extending to axilla

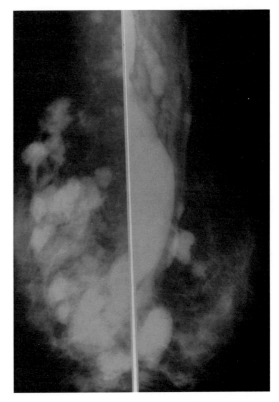

FIGURE 12-11
Subcutaneous silicone injections.
Dense, irregular, variably sized
masses scattered bilaterally, consistent with previous subcutaneous silicone injections.

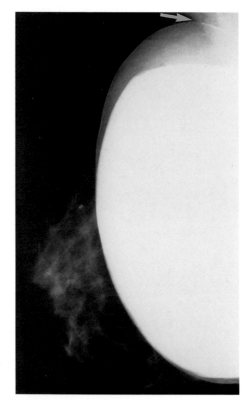

FIGURE 12-12
Subglandular (prepectoral), double-lumen (outer saline, inner silicone) implant, right mediolateral oblique view. Double-lumen implants are characterized by density differences, seen superiorly in this patient. Pectoral muscle seen "diving" (*arrow*) behind implant (when implant is prepectoral).

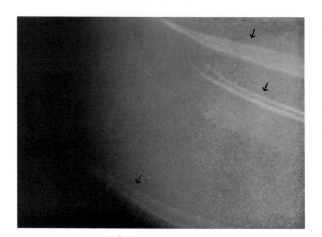

FIGURE 12-13
Saline implant with wrinkles (*arrows*).

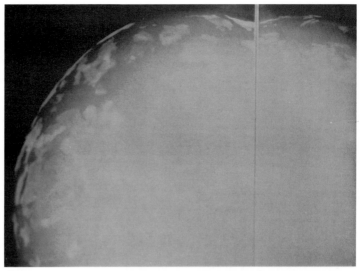

A

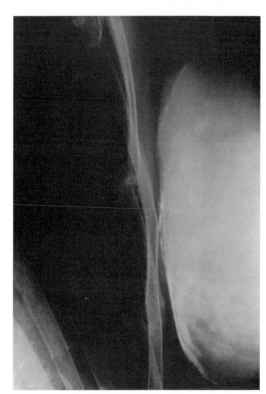

FIGURE 12-14
(A) Coarse capsular calcifications. These calcifications generally develop in the fibrous capsule after capsular contraction. (B) Capsular calcifications. Chest wall view done to demonstrate posterior portion of implant. Chest wall view is done with aluminum filter, no compression, and 38 to 42 kV.

B

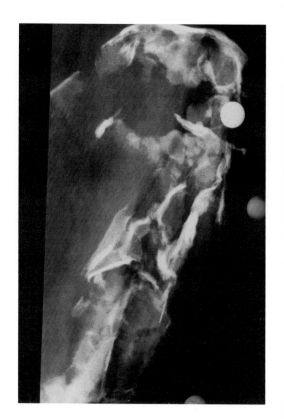

FIGURE 12-15
Dense capsular calcification seen
on follow-up after implant removal.

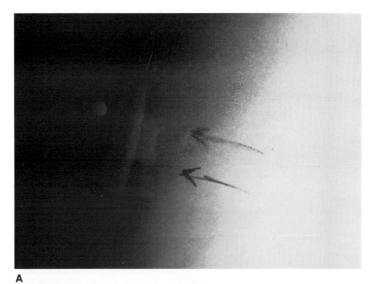

A

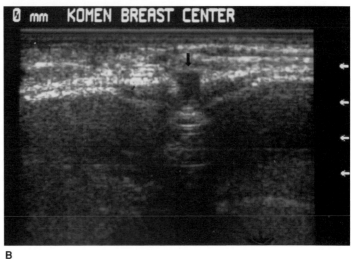

B

FIGURE 12-16
Saline implant with palpable port. (**A**) Metallic BB (*arrows*). (**B**) Rectangular hypoechoic area (*arrow*) corresponding to area of palpable concern.

Implant Complications

KEY FACTS

- Gel bleed
    - A semipermeable silicone outer shell surrounds inner silicone or saline.
    - Depending on the extent of cross-linking of the silicone elastomer shell, implants are characterized by low or high grades of gel bleed. Silicone or saline actually bleeds out of intact implants because of the semipermeable nature of the shell.
    - The immune system of women with intact implants is exposed to variable amounts of silicone soon after augmentation.
    - On MRI, gel bleed is reflected by the filling in of wrinkles ("keyholes").
- Capsule
    - As foreign bodies, implants are walled off by the formation of a fibrous capsule.
    - This capsule (bands of fibrous tissue) forms in all women with implants.
    - In some women, the capsule remains soft.
    - In other women, the capsule starts to strangulate the implant, leading to various degrees of encapsulation.
    - With encapsulation, implants become hard and difficult to move (displaced implant views may be difficult to obtain) and no longer feel or look natural.
    - Encapsulation is apparent mammographically: the implants become round on MLO views.
    - Many implant modifications were attempts to deal with capsular contraction. For instance, textured implants were introduced under the theory that the rough surface would create a disturbance of the fibrous tissue in the capsule, preventing contraction. Subpectoral placement was introduced in hopes that the muscular movement over the implant would serve to disrupt capsule formation.
    - Closed capsulotomy: physical compression of the capsule so as to break the capsule, softening the feel of the implant. Complications of closed capsulotomies include bleeding, implant rupture, and, for the plastic surgeon, injury to the ulnar collateral ligament ("gamekeeper's thumb").
    - Open capsulotomy: surgical removal of capsule
- Intracapsular rupture
    - Silicone is free within the capsule formed by the patient.
    - This type of rupture cannot usually be identified mammographically.
    - "Linguini sign" on magnetic resonance imaging
    - It has been suggested that with time (more than 10 years), the shell of many implants may be nonexistent and the silicone or saline is contained only by the woman's native capsule.

- Extracapsular rupture
  - Silicone is free and found outside the implant and capsule.
  - Silicone can be seen migrating to the axillary lymph nodes.
- Autoimmune disorders
  - No definitive proof of a relation between silicone and autoimmune disorders

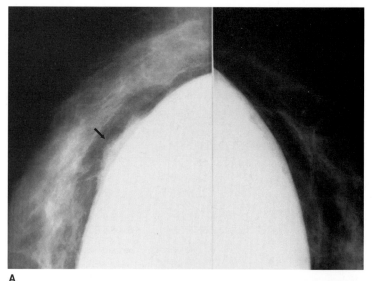

A

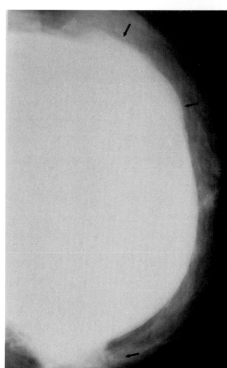

FIGURE 12-17
Extracapsular rupture. (**A**) Irregular area of high density (*arrow*) associated with lateral portion of right implant. (**B**) Irregular areas of high density (*arrows*) surrounding implant. In some patients, silicone is seen extending to the axillary lymph nodes.

B

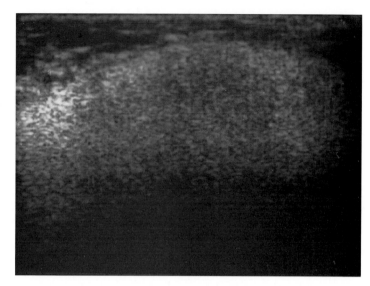

FIGURE 12-18
Implant rupture. "Snowstorm" appearance described for extraluminal silicone. Irregular hypoechoic masses on ultrasound have also been described with implant rupture.

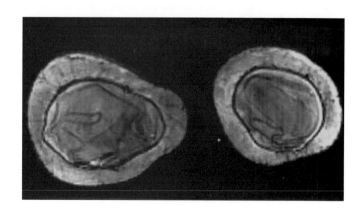

FIGURE 12-19
Implant rupture. Linguini sign on magnetic resonance imaging. Presumably, the implant shell is floating in silicone.

Reduction Mammoplasty

KEY FACTS

- Medical indications for reduction
    - Extra weight may lead to respiratory compromise.
    - Alterations in posture may lead to kyphosis.
    - Back, anterior thoracic, or breast pain
    - Shoulder strap marks from bra
    - Intertrigal infections (inframammary fold)
    - Psychosocial issues
- Understanding the surgical approach used facilitates understanding mammographic changes.
    - Circumareolar incision (keyhole incision)—attention to maintaining vascular supply
    - Sagittal incision from areola to inframammary fold (6 o'clock position)
    - At the inframammary fold, horizontal incisions are made to create two flaps (lateral and medial).
    - Tissue is scooped out.
    - The nipple and areola must be repositioned. In older women, the ducts can be transected behind the nipple and the nipple–areolar complex moved in isolation (transplantation). In younger women who may want to breast feed in the future, the duct–nipple connection can be maintained so that the nipple–areolar complex is moved with the subareolar ducts attached (transposition).
- Complications
    - Avascular necrosis of nipple–areolar complex, skin, or breast parenchyma
    - Wound infections (unusual)
    - Loss of sensation around nipple area
    - Fat necrosis
    - Hypertrophic scarring
    - Inadequate or overreduction
    - "Bottoming out"
- Mammographic findings on MLO views
    - Redistribution inferiorly and swirling pattern of tissue
    - Tilting or elevation of nipple—may become more striking with time ("bottoming out")
    - Skin thickening along sagittal scar

- Mammographic findings on MLO and CC views
  - Nonanatomically distributed islands of glandular tissue
  - Fibrotic bands in subareolar area (nonanatomic in appearance)
  - Fat necrosis, oil cysts (single or multiple), dystrophic calcifications
  - Skin thickening
  - Disruption of subareolar ducts after nipple transplantation
  - Epidermal inclusion cysts

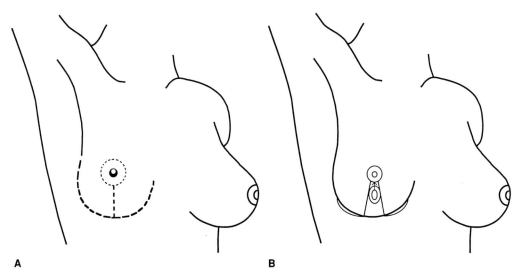

A   B

FIGURE 12-20   (**A**) Circumareolar and sagittal incisions (6 o'clock) to the inframammary fold, then a horizontal incision is made, creating medial and lateral flaps. Tissue is then scooped out inferiorly. (**B**) Nipple–areola complex must be repositioned superiorly, either isolated from the subareolar ducts (transplantation) or with the subareolar ducts still attached (transposition).

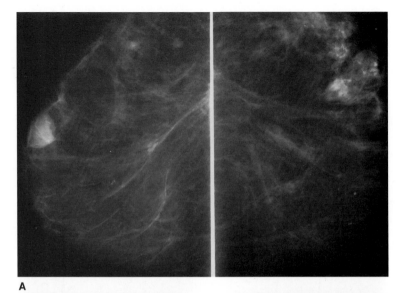

A

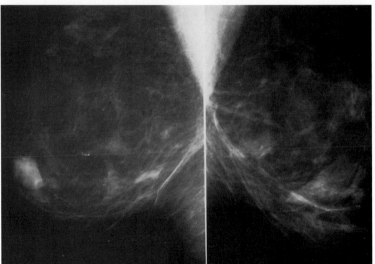

B

FIGURE 12-21
Reduction mammoplasty. (**A**) Right
and left craniocaudal views. Asymmetric islands of breast tissue in a
nonanatomic distribution. Swirling
of tissue. Small, scattered, coarse,
dense, benign-type calcifications bilaterally. (**B**) Right and left mediolateral oblique views. Swirling of
tissue inferiorly, islands of tissue in
a nonanatomic distribution. Small,
scattered, coarse, dense, benign-
type calcifications bilaterally.

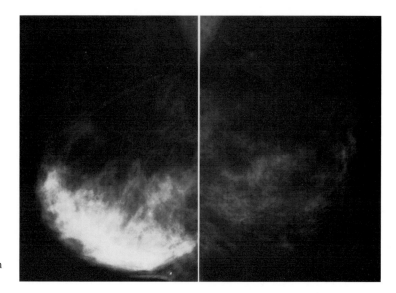

FIGURE 12-22
Reduction mammoplasty. Right and
left mediolateral oblique views.
Asymmetric tissue (right greater than
left) inferiorly displaced.

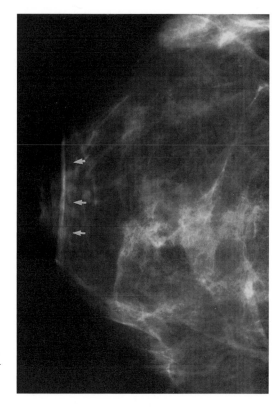

FIGURE 12-23
Reduction mammoplasty. Right
craniocaudal view. Horizontal band
(*arrows*) in subareolar area (nonanatomic) and islands of tissue in a
nonanatomic distribution.

Hormone Replacement

KEY FACTS

- Clinical
  - Estrogen stimulates proliferation of ductal system and periductal stroma.
  - Progesterone counteracts some of the proliferative effects of estrogen and promotes lobular development.
  - Estrogen replacement therapy is advocated for treating postmenopausal symptoms, preventing osteoporosis, and providing potential cardiovascular benefits.
  - Breast pain, fullness, masses, and nodularity may develop in women on estrogen.
  - Studies on associated breast cancer risk, inconclusive
- Mammography
  - Diffuse increase in density of breast tissue
  - Multifocal, asymmetric densities
  - Cyst formation
  - Changes in up to 24% of patients placed on exogenous estrogen
  - May be related to duration of treatment
  - More common in women on estrogen and progesterone (as opposed to estrogen alone)

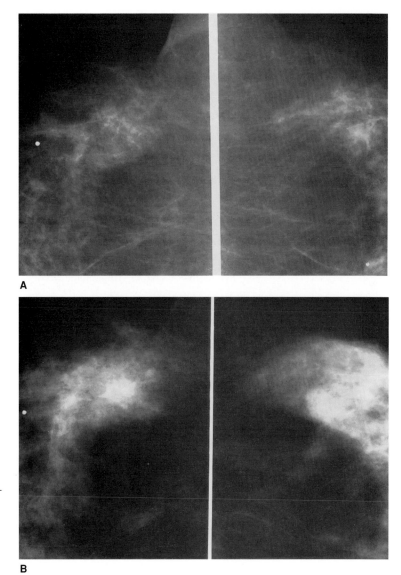

FIGURE 12-24
Estrogen effect. (**A**) Right and left craniocaudal (CC) views. Pre-estrogen. (**B**) Right and left CC views. Increased tissue and tissue density developing during first year of exogenous estrogen use. Some patients develop single or multiple cysts.

Miscellaneous

KEY FACTS

- Weight changes
  - Weight increase may result in mammographically perceptible breast size changes, breast tissue dispersal, and increases in the amount of fatty tissue.
  - Weight loss may result in a mammographically perceptible decrease in breast size, breast tissue aggregation, and loss of fatty tissue.
- Chemotherapy
  - May result in decreases in the amount of tissue
- Tamoxifen
  - Antiestrogenic and estrogenic action
  - Tissue may decrease in density; this agent has been used in Europe to treat symptoms of severe, symptomatic fibrocystic change.
- Pacemakers
  - May be partially or completely seen on MLO views superimposed on pectoral muscle
  - If the pacemaker is removed, coarse calcification of the pacemaker cavity may develop.
  - If the pacemaker is removed, remaining pacemaker wires may be seen.
- Dacron central line cuff
  - For Hickman catheter placement, a 4″ to 6″ subcutaneous tunnel is made and a Dacron cuff is used to anchor the catheter to the subcutaneous tissue.
  - When the Hickman catheter is pulled out, the cuff remains in place and may be seen on both MLO (more common) and CC views.
  - May be palpable
  - Irregular mass (which may contain air) around cuff may indicate abcess formation (P. J. Dempsey, MD, personal communication)
- Subcutaneous air after pneumothorax or chest tube
- Lactation
  - Increases breast tissue density diffusely
  - Prominent subareolar ducts seen ultrasonographically
- Premenstrual edema
  - In some women, there can be significant density increases premenstrually, presumably related to fluid accumulation and retention.
  - Enlargement of pre-existing cysts

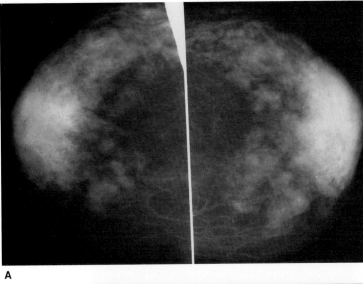

A

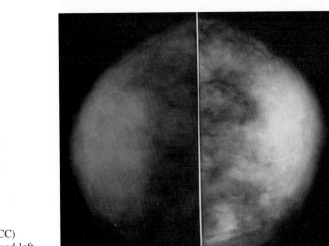

FIGURE 12-25

Weight loss. (**A**) Right and left craniocaudal (CC) screening views before weight loss. (**B**) Right and left CC screening views after a 40-lb weight loss. Decreased breast size, reduction in fatty tissue, confluence of glandular tissue.

B

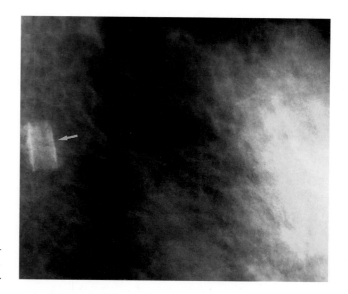

FIGURE 12-26
Hickman Dacron cuff. Cuff used to anchor central line. When the line is pulled, the cuff remains in place (*arrow*). May be palpable. More commonly seen on mediolateral oblique view superimposed on pectoral muscle. In some women, can also be seen medially on craniocaudal views.

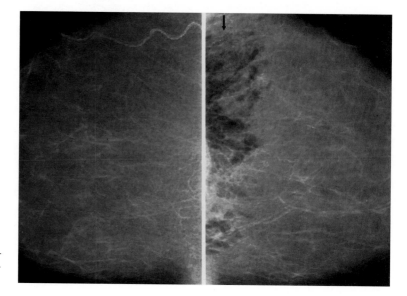

FIGURE 12-27
Subcutaneous emphysema. Right and left craniocaudal views. Subcutaneous air (*arrow*), left breast posteriorly.

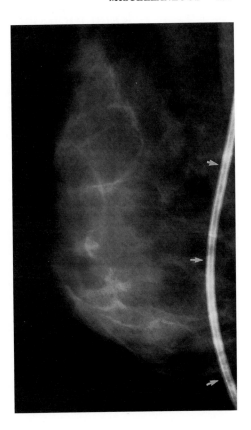

FIGURE 12-28
Shunt tubing (*arrows*). Tubing superimposed on right breast tissue posteriorly.

BIBLIOGRAPHY

Berkowitz JE, Gatewood OMB, Goldblum LE, Gayler BW. Hormonal replacement therapy: mammographic manifestations. Radiology 1990;174:199–201

Beyer GA, Thorsen MK, Shaffer KA, Walker AP. Mammographic appearance of the retained Dacron cuff of a Hickman catheter. AJR 1990;155:1204

Cardenosa G, Eklund GW. Breast parenchymal change following treatment with tamoxifen [letter]. Breast Dis 1992;5:55–58

Cardenosa G, Eklund GW. Imaging the altered breast. In Taveras JM, Ferrucci JT (eds). Radiology: diagnosis, imaging, intervention. Philadelphia, JB Lippincott 1993

DeBruhl ND, Gorczyca DP, Ahn CY, Shaw WW, Bassett LW. Silicone breast implants: US evaluation. Radiology 1993;189:95–98

Dershaw DD. Mammography in patients with breast cancer treated by breast conservation (lumpectomy with or without radiation). AJR 1995;164:309–316

Destouet JM, Monsees BS, Oser RF, et al. Screening mammography in 350 women with breast implants: prevalence and findings of implant complications. AJR 1992;159:973–978

Everson LI, Parantainen H, Detlie T, et al. Diagnosis of breast implant rupture: imaging findings and relative efficacies of imaging techniques. AJR 1994;163:57–60

Fajardo LL, Bessen SC. Epidermal inclusion cysts after reduction mammoplasty. Radiology 1993;186:103–106

Fajardo LL, Roberts CC, Hunt KR. Mammographic surveillance of breast cancer patients: should the mastectomy site be imaged? AJR 1993;161:953–955

Ganott MA, Harris KM, Ilkanipour ZS, Costa-Greco MA. Augmentation mammoplasty: normal and abnormal findings with mammography and US. RadioGraphics 1992;12:281–295

Gorczyca DP, DeBruhl ND, Mund DF, Bassett LW. Linguini sign at MR imaging: does it represent the collapsed silicone implant shell? Radiology 1994;191:576–577

Harris KM, Ganott MA, Shestak KC, Losken HW, Tobon H. Silicone implant rupture: detection with US. Radiology 1993;187:761–768

Mendelson EB. Imaging the postsurgical breast. Semin Ultrasound CT MR 1989;10:154–170

Mendelson EB. Evaluation of the postoperative breast. Radiol Clin North Am 1992;30:107–138

Mendelson EB, Tobin CE. Imaging the breast after surgery and radiation therapy. RSNA Categorical Course in Breast Imaging Syllabus 1995, pp 175–184

Miller CL, Feig SA, Fox JW. Mammographic changes after reduction mammoplasty. AJR 1987;149:35–38

Mund DF, Farria DM, Gorczyca DP, et al. MR imaging of the breast in patients with silicone-gel implants: spectrum of findings. AJR 1993;161:773–778

Ricciardi I, Ianniruberto A. Tamoxifen-induced regression of benign breast lesions. Obstet Gynecol 1979;51:80–84

Rissanen TJ, Makarainen HP, Mattila SI, Lindholm EL, Heikkinen MI, Kiviniemi HO. Breast cancer recurrence after mastectomy: diagnosis with mammography and US. Radiology 1993;188:463–467

Rosculet KA, Ikeda DM, Forrest ME, et al. Ruptured gel-filled silicone breast implants: sonographic findings in 19 cases. AJR 1992;159:711–716

Stomper PC, Van Voorhis BJ, Ravnikar VA, Meyer JE. Mammographic changes associated with postmenopausal hormone replacement therapy: a longitudinal study. Radiology 1990;174:487–490

Breast Imaging Companion
by Gilda Cardenosa
Lippincott-Raven Publishers, Philadelphia © 1997

Chapter 13

THE MALE BREAST

Imaging the Male Breast

KEY FACTS

- The initial evaluation of male patients presenting with breast-related symptoms includes craniocaudal and mediolateral oblique views of the symptomatic breast. Contralateral breast images may be done for comparison.

- The compression paddle used for most female patients makes it difficult for the technologist to hold the male breast in place as compression is applied. Technologists may find it difficult to slide their hand out from under the compression paddle without scraping their knuckles. For this reason, some equipment manufacturers provide a narrow paddle (approximately half the width of the compression paddles used for most female patients).

- As in female patients, diagnostic views (eg, spot compression, spot magnification, tangential, rolled) may be indicated if an abnormality is detected on initial views.

- In male patients, predominantly fatty tissue, prominent pectoral muscles, and a small nipple are mammographic characteristics. When evaluating films and discussing cases, look at all the information provided on the film (eg, patient name, age, date of study).

- Male breast tissue contains major subareolar ducts with little secondary branching.

- Because lobular units are rare (approximately one in 1000 men), lobular lesions (fibroadenoma, sclerosing adenosis) are unusual.

- Although only two entities are discussed in this chapter, all lesions described in female patients can occur in male patients. However, the incidence in men is significantly lower, particularly for the lobular-derived lesions.

Gynecomastia

KEY FACTS

- Clinical
  - Enlargement of the male breast: subareolar ducts develop secondary branching and there is proliferation of the surrounding stroma
  - Unilateral or bilateral, symmetric or asymmetric
  - Early: subareolar with concentric distribution; eccentric masses are of concern
  - Idiopathic or related to estrogen excess (hormone imbalance)
  - Physiologic: neonate (placental estrogens); pubertal (60% to 70% of adolescent males; breast enlargement and tenderness may be asymmetric); elderly (related to decreases in plasma testosterone levels)
  - Underlying diseases with estrogen excess: testicular tumors; nontesticular tumors (skin, adrenocortical, lung, hepatocellular carcinoma); liver cirrhosis; endocrine (hypo- and hyperthyroidism); nutritional deprivation (in some men gynecomastia develops after a period of nutritional deprivation, when normal feeding is resumed [refeeding gynecomastia]).
  - Androgen deficiency: aging; primary testicular failure, hypogonadism (Klinefelter's syndrome); secondary testicular failure (trauma, orchitis, cryptorchidism, irradiation, hydrocele); renal failure
  - Drugs: estrogenic activity (anabolic steroids, digitalis, heroin, marijuana); inhibition of testosterone action or synthesis (cimetidine, diazepam, phenytoin, spironolactone, vincristine, methotrexate); idiopathic mechanism (furosemide, isoniazid, methyldopa, nifedipine, reserpine, theophylline, proscar, verapamil)
  - Systemic disorders associated with gynecomastia—mechanism unknown: nonneoplastic diseases of the lung; trauma to chest wall; AIDS
  - Most men present with a subareolar mass, tenderness, or both.

- Mammography
  - Early: nodular pattern—increased tissue focally in subareolar area
  - Late: fibrous phase—tissue radiating out from nipple (triangular)
  - Diffuse glandular pattern
  - Unilateral or asymmetric, 72%
  - If classic gynecomastia is seen with no microcalcifications or eccentric mass, biopsy may be averted unless the patient is symptomatic.

- Histology
  - Male breast contains major ducts only.
  - Early: proliferation of ducts and surrounding connective tissue; reversible if source of estrogens is withdrawn
  - Late: fibrosis and hyalinization; ducts become less prominent; once fibrosis occurs, process is irreversible

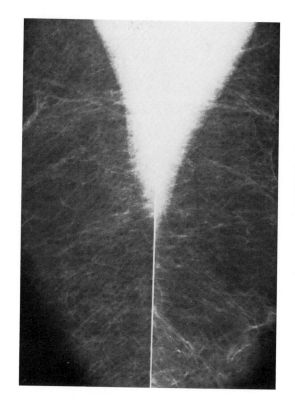

FIGURE 13-1
Prominent fatty tissue, male breast.

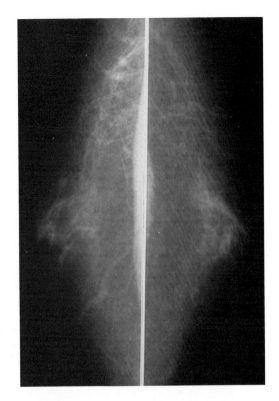

FIGURE 13-2
Gynecomastia. Craniocaudal views
showing small amount of subareolar
tissue (left greater than right).

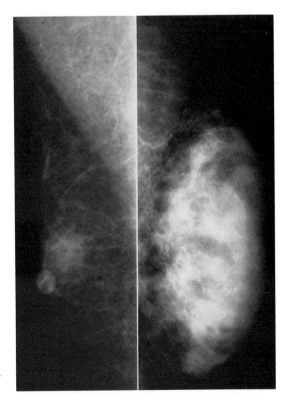

FIGURE 13-3
Gynecomastia. Mediolateral
oblique views with strikingly
asymmetric gynecomastia. Minor
development of glandular tissue,
right subareolar area. Diffuse glandular pattern on the left.

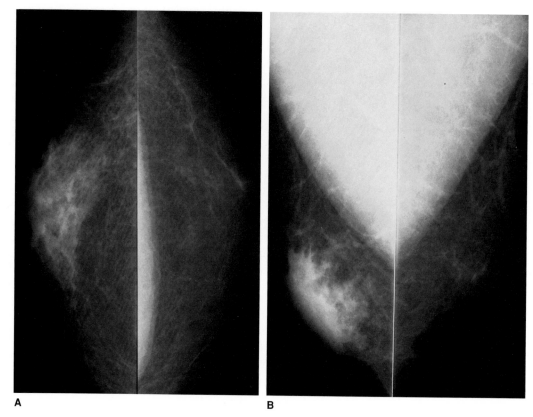

A   B

FIGURE 13-4   Gynecomastia. (**A**) Craniocaudal and (**B**) mediolateral oblique views. Asymmetric development of dense glandular tissue, right subareolar area. Predominantly fatty tissue on the left. Prominent pectoral muscles.

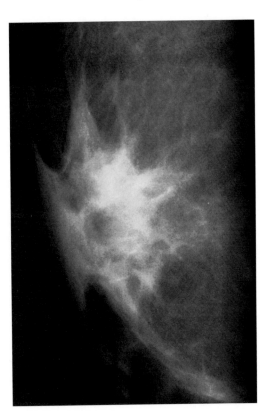

FIGURE 13-5
Gynecomastia. Micro-focus (0.1 mm)
spot magnification view of the subareolar area demonstrates normal fibroglandular pattern with no underlying
mass or calcifications.

Male Breast Cancer

KEY FACTS

- Clinical
  - Less than 0.5% of all breast cancers
  - Older mean age (64) than for female breast cancers
  - Increased incidence in men with Klinefelter's syndrome, mumps orchitis after age 20, Jews, African-Americans
  - Probably unrelated to gynecomastia
  - 85% infiltrating ductal carcinomas (not otherwise specified); 5% each intraductal or papillary; lobular carcinoma extremely rare
  - Painless, hard mass
  - 25% of patients have nipple discharge or ulceration.
  - Prognosis depends on lymph node status and size of tumor at time of diagnosis.

- Mammography
  - Microcalcifications (in up to 30% of male breast cancers)
  - Mass: well circumscribed to spiculated

- Histology
  - No different from findings for female breast cancer types

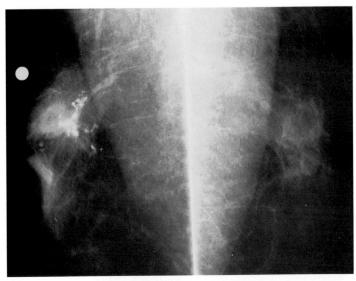

A

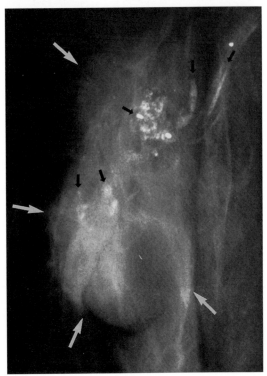

FIGURE 13-6

Infiltrating ductal carcinoma (not otherwise specified [NOS]) with ductal carcinoma in situ (DCIS) in male patient. (**A**) Mediolateral oblique views demonstrating mass with associated calcifications on the right. Metallic BB indicate presence of a palpable mass. Minor gynecomastia is present on the left. Prominent pectoral muscles. (**B**) Microfocus (0.1 mm) spot magnification view demonstrating the mass and associated calcifications. The mass (*white arrows*) reflects underlying infiltrating ductal carcinoma (NOS), and the calcifications (*black arrows*) represent multifocal DCIS (mixed nuclear grade).

B

BIBLIOGRAPHY

Chantra PK, So GJ, Wollman JS, Bassett LW. Mammography of the male breast. AJR 1995; 164:853–858

Cooper RA, Gunter BA, Ramamurthy L. Mammography in men. Radiology 1994;191: 651–656

Breast Imaging Companion
by Gilda Cardenosa
Lippincott-Raven Publishers, Philadelphia © 1997

Chapter 14

INTERVENTIONAL PROCEDURES

Preoperative Needle Localizations

KEY FACTS

- Indications
  - Nonpalpable, clinically occult lesions
  - In some women with palpable lesions, to ensure excision of the lesion and a one-to-one correlation between mammographic and clinical lesion
- Mammography, ultrasound, and stereotactic systems can be used to guide pre-operative localizations.
- Methods
  - Skin localizations—unless the lesion is close to the skin surface (within 1 cm), skin localizations are imprecise, leading to the excision of large amounts of tissue to be sure of encompassing the area of concern
  - Dye method (methylene blue, alcian blue)—after verification of needle position, dye is injected; as needle is pulled out, track of dye is left. Some have suggested that diffusion of dye leads to excision of larger amounts of tissue than needed. However, in our experience, if a minute amount of dye is used (approximately 0.2 cc), not much diffusion is seen. There has been one report of methylene blue affecting estrogen-receptor assays.
  - Needles and needle–wire combinations; latter preferred
  - Injection of dye can be combined with wire placement. The dye serves as a back-up should anything happen to the wire during surgery.
  - Methods described for lesions seen in only one view are beyond the scope of this book. See the articles in the bibliography by Kopans, Waitzkin, Linetsky and colleagues and Pollack for more detailed descriptions of these methods.
- Needle–wire combinations come in different lengths (eg, 3, 5, 7, 9, 11, and 15 cm).
  - Hookwire system: modified hookwire includes a (2 cm long) reinforced wire segment 1.2 cm from the hook
  - J-wire: flexible, J-shaped wire can be retracted back into needle if repositioning is needed
  - retractable barb (Hawkins)
- Three decisions: type of needle–wire, needle length, and approach
- Approaches: anteroposterior and parallel to the chest wall
- Compression paddles for localizations
  - Regular-sized compression paddle with fenestration and alphanumeric grid most common
  - Regular-sized compression paddle with multiple holes; may require repositioning if lesion is not under one of the openings

- Spot compression paddle with multiple holes is particularly useful in women with small breasts or with a lesion high in the breast (toward axilla), far posterior, or in the subareolar area. This paddle affords the benefits of a spot compression paddle: maximal compression and ability to reach up or back further (attaining sufficient compression and immobilization) than with a regular compression paddle.

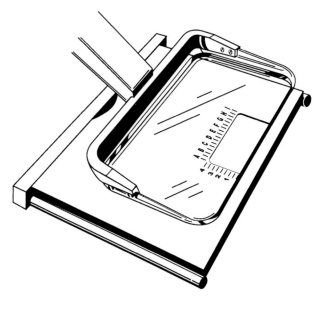

FIGURE 14-1
Compression paddle with fenestration and alphanumeric grid used for most localizations and mammographically guided cyst aspirations.

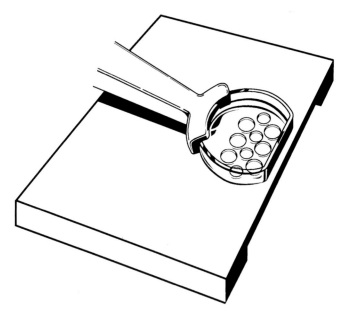

FIGURE 14-2
Multiple-hole spot compression paddle. Particularly useful when optimal immobilization may not be obtainable with the regular compression paddle—specifically, lesions high in the breast (toward axilla), far posterior, or subareolar in location. Also useful in women with a small breast. If the lesion is not under one of the openings, repositioning may be necessary.

Anteroposterior Needle Localization Approach

KEY FACTS

- Radiologist must extrapolate lesion location from images of a compressed breast pulled away from the body to a decompressed breast in its natural position.

- Needle is advanced in breast blindly toward the chest wall.

- Orthogonal images are obtained to determine the relation of the needle to the lesion.

- If the needle is not within 1 cm of the lesion in orthogonal views, you may want to reposition the needle. Use the images to help determine the direction the needle needs to go.

- After the needle is repositioned, orthogonal images are done again. The needle may need to be repositioned several times before placement is acceptable (within 1 cm of lesion).

- When needle positioning is acceptable, the wire is engaged and films are obtained to establish final wire positioning.

- Although some have suggested a higher complication rate (primarily pneumothorax, although wire migration may be more common with this approach also) with an anteroposterior approach, this has not been studied systematically. If the needle is advanced in the breast carefully, this is a safe and acceptable method of localizing breast lesions.

- Because this method requires serial approximations (the needle may have to be repositioned several times before the lesion is localized appropriately), it may be more time-consuming and harder to teach and learn.

- Complications (unusual)
  - Bleeding
  - Pneumothorax
  - Migration of wire (in breast or to distant sites)

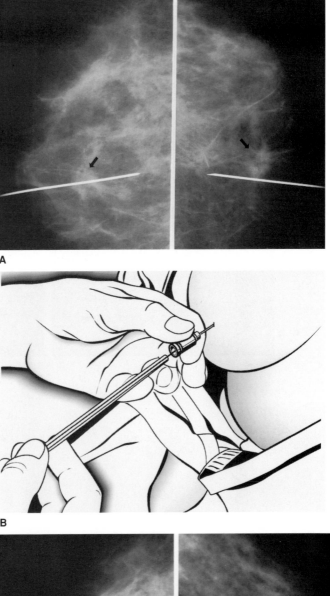

A

B

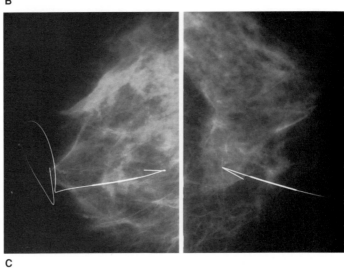

C

FIGURE 14-3

(A) Anteroposterior localization approach. 90° lateral and craniocaudal (CC) views back to back obtained after needle placement. Acceptable needle placement; needle within 1 cm of spiculated mass (*arrows*) on orthogonal views. If at this point the needle is not within 1 cm of the lesion, repositioning is undertaken. (B) The wire is passed through the needle. The needle is removed and orthogonal views are done to verify final wire positioning. Patient sitting with breast uncompressed. (C) Anteroposterior localization approach. 90° lateral and CC views back to back obtained after wire placement. Reinforced wire segment is alongside a spiculated mass on orthogonal views.

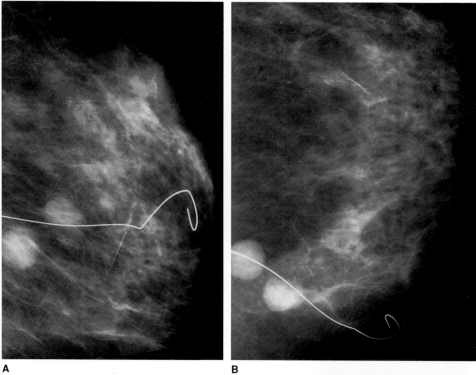

A   B

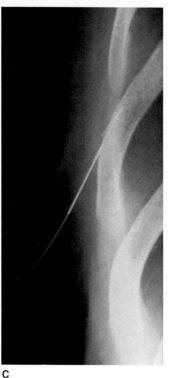

FIGURE 14-4
(**A**) Anteroposterior localization approach. 90° lateral view after
wire placement. Two masses being localized. What is the problem? (**B**) Anteroposterior localization approach. Craniocaudal (CC)
view after wire placement. The wire is within 1 cm of both
masses in orthogonal views, but where is the hook? What can you
do at this point (patient is breathing OK)? (**C**) Chest wall view.
Wire in close proximity to a rib. Care must be exercised as the
needle–wire is advanced in the breast. This approach is more difficult to teach and learn because it requires extrapolation of the lesion location in the breast from CC and 90° lateral views (during
which the breast is pulled out away from the body and compressed) to the breast in an uncompressed, natural state. In experienced hands, however, this localization approach can be safe and
accurate. Two fibroadenomas on histology.

C

Parallel to the Chest Wall

KEY FACTS

NEEDLE LOCALIZATION APPROACH

- Approach selection
  - Established by reviewing orthogonal views (craniocaudal [CC] and 90° lateral views) to determine shortest skin-to-lesion distance
  - If the lesion is closest to the lateral portion of the breast (CC view), the alphanumeric paddle is used to compress the lateral portion of the breast and a 90° lateromedial view is done.
  - If the lesion is closest to the medial portion of the breast (CC view), the alphanumeric paddle is used to compress the medial portion of the breast and a 90° mediolateral view is done.
  - If the lesion is closest to the top of the breast (90° lateral view), the alphanumeric paddle is used to compress the upper portion of the breast and a CC view is done.
  - If the lesion is closest to the bottom of the breast (90° lateral view), the alphanumeric paddle is used to compress the inferior portion of the breast and a caudocranial (reverse CC) view is done.

- Needle length
  - Established by measuring the distance from expected skin entry site to lesion
  - Needle must be long enough to go beyond the lesion by at least 1 cm. If the needle is too long, it can be pulled out as much as needed before engaging the wire. However, if the needle is short of the lesion, nothing much can be done other than to start all over. It is always preferable to err on the side of selecting a long needle.

- Written consent obtained

- Pitfalls
  - Selecting the wrong approach; not using the shortest distance to reach the lesion. The surgeon should not have to go across quadrants to remove a clinically occult lesion.
  - Using a too-short needle
  - Vasovagal reactions—this is a stressful time for patients and they are usually fasting, so be prepared to handle vasovagal reactions. Some use atropine routinely (0.6 mg IM or IV) to prevent vasovagal reaction (contraindicated in patients with glaucoma).

PROCEDURE

- With approach and needle length selected, the patient is positioned. For purposes of discussion, let us say the lesion to be localized is closest to the superior skin surface on the 90° lateral view and we are using a modified needle–wire system.

(text continues on the next page)

Parallel to the Chest Wall *(Continued)*

- Using the alphanumeric fenestrated paddle for compression, a CC view is obtained to establish lesion coordinates (patient is sitting during procedure).
  - Skin is cleansed with alcohol wipe and 1% lidocaine is used to raise a skin wheal. If lidocaine is injected slowly, the stinging sensation described by patients may be minimized. Use of lidocaine is optional.

- Using the collimator cross-hairs, a shadow of the lesion's coordinates is cast on the breast. The needle (we work with the needle alone at this point; the wire is pulled out of the needle and set aside) is angled so that the tip can be placed at the intersection of the cross-hairs and then straightened.

- Holding the needle with the thumb and index finger, spread the other fingers apart away from the needle so you can see the needle hub shadow and its relation to the cross-hairs. Otherwise, the hand casts a shadow, making it impossible to see the cross-hairs. Laser lights are available on some units, but in our opinion these are not ideal: they make some of the described maneuvers difficult if not impossible.

- The needle is advanced all the way into the breast in one rapid motion. Don't worry about depth: the worst that will happen is that you approach and feel the bucky on the contralateral side of the breast. As you approach the contralateral skin, the patient may experience discomfort.

- The cross-hairs are moved out of the way and a film is obtained. If the hub of the needle, needle shaft, and lesion are superimposed and you selected a long enough needle, the lesion is skewered.

- Compression is released, taking care that the needle hub does not become engaged on the edge of the compression paddle, as this may result in the inadvertent removal of the needle.

- Using a spot compression paddle (using the regular compression paddle may preclude adequate access to the needle for manipulation—the distance between paddle and bucky can be minimal, particularly in women with small breasts) the breast is compressed in the orthogonal direction. In this example, a 90° lateral view is obtained to establish where along the course of the needle the lesion is located.

- The tip of the needle should be 1 cm beyond the lesion, ensuring that the reinforced segment of the modified wire is placed within or alongside the lesion.

- If needle location is appropriate (in this example, the needle is superimposed on the lesion in the CC view and the lesion is along the course of the needle on the 90° lateral view), methylene blue can be injected, if desired, as a backup for the surgeon, and the wire is engaged.

- The needle is removed, ensuring that the wire is not advanced or pulled out with needle removal.

- A follow-up film is obtained to document final wire positioning.

- The orthogonal views obtained during localization (CC with the needle hub and shaft superimposed on the lesion and 90° lateral view with wire in place) are reviewed with the surgeon. The amount of tissue and any relevant particulars (eg, avoid frozen section, multicentricity) can be discussed.

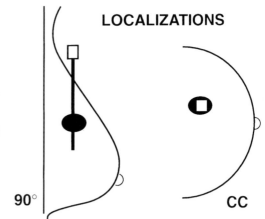

FIGURE 14-7
It is important to see the needle associated with the lesion in orthogonal views. In this case (lesion approached from the superior portion of the breast), the needle hub and shaft are superimposed on the lesion in the craniocaudal view; if a long enough needle is used, the lesion is skewered. This is confirmed on the lateral view: the needle is seen going through the lesion.

FIGURE 14-8
In this case, the wrong approach and needle length were selected. The lesion is inferiorly located, so a superior approach is unacceptable. Although the hub and shaft of the needle are superimposed on the lesion in the craniocaudal view, the needle is not long enough to reach the lesion. The needle must be associated with the lesion in both views—if not, something is wrong (eg, approach, needle length, lesion on one view does not correspond to what is being looked at on second view). When the needle is not associated with the lesion on orthogonal views, stop and reassess the situation. Do not engage the hookwire.

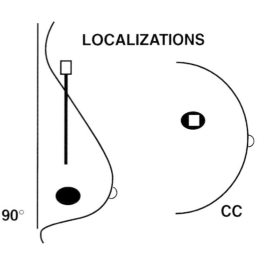

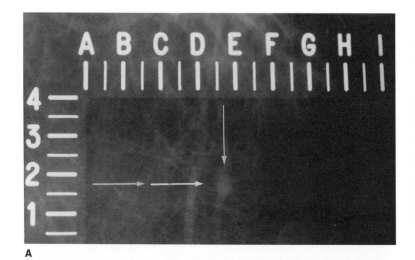

A

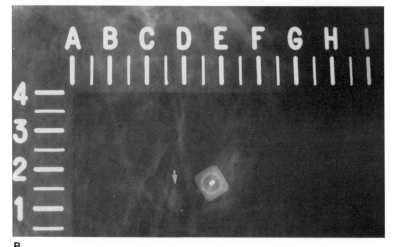

FIGURE 14-9
(**A**) Small mass at D.75 and 1.75.
(**B**) Needle in at D.75 and 1.75, but
needle hub and shaft are not superimposed on mass. Mass (*arrow*) is
now at C.5 and 1.25. Patient moved
between the taking of **A** and needle
insertion. Marking the corners of
the fenestration on the patient's
skin can alert you that the patient
moved after the initial image. In
this patient, a second needle was in-
serted at the new lesion coordinates.

B

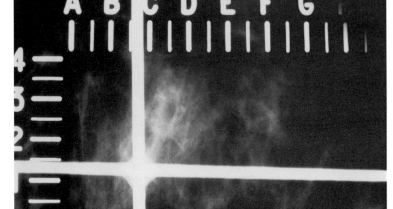

FIGURE 14-10
If after needle insertion you forget
to move the collimator cross-hairs,
evaluation on this orthogonal view
is precluded (lesion, needle hub and
shaft not visualized).

Specimen Radiography

KEY FACTS

- Obtained for all (eg, microcalcifications, masses, areas of parenchymal asymmetry, architectural distortion) breast biopsies done after needle localization
- Purposes
  - Verifies removal of the lesion localized
  - Can be used to guide the pathologist to the location of the lesion in the specimen. We place a needle through the lesion so that we are sure the area of radiologic concern is evaluated histologically.
  - To verify that the wire has been removed from the breast. If the wire is not seen in the specimen, we ask about its whereabouts when we call the surgeon to let her or him know that the lesion has been excised, and we document what is said.
  - May be able to assess proximity to margins (remember, however, that a radiograph is a two-dimensional representation of a three-dimensional structure)
  - To detect additional, unsuspected lesions
  - As a learning tool: particularly useful during radiology/pathology correlation sessions in learning about lesion morphology and correlation with histologic findings
- Procedure
  - Done on mammographic unit or dedicated specimen radiography unit
  - Specimen is compressed.
  - Two magnified (1.6 to 1.8 $\times$) views are done (one for our records, one for the pathologist).
  - Lowest possible kV (22 kV); mAs 4–5
  - Communicate with operating room and surgeon as to whether the lesion has been excised or not, if there is proximity to margins, and the appropriateness of frozen section and so forth. If the wire is not in the specimen, ask about the wire.
  - Our impressions are also communicated to the pathologist.

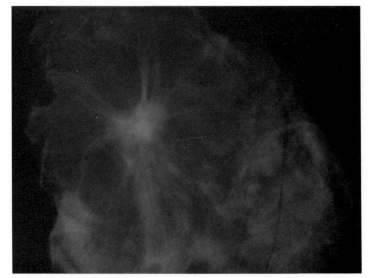

FIGURE 14-11
Specimen radiograph after localization shown in Figure 14-3. Excision of spiculated mass verified. Location of the mass in the specimen can be marked for the pathologist (we use a needle). Special specimen containers with localizing grids are commercially available, but they are expensive. Infiltrating ductal carcinoma, well differentiated.

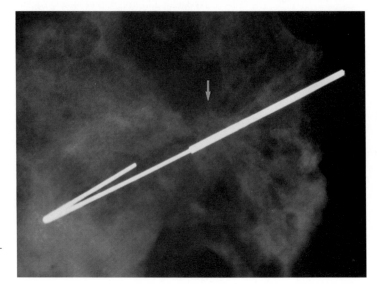

FIGURE 14-12
Specimen radiograph following localization shown in Figure 14-6. What would you accept as a diagnosis for this? Tubular carcinoma histologically. Did you consider radial scar?

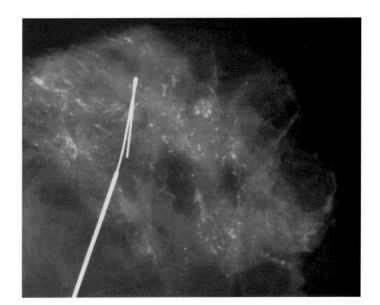

FIGURE 14-13
Extensive area of microcalcifications on the specimen. Pleomorphic calcifications with amorphous and linear forms predominating. It is important to communicate with the surgeon and pathologist that there is probably tumor extending to the margins (confirmed histologically). DCIS, predominantly poorly differentiated.

Paraffin Block Radiography

KEY FACTS

- After a biopsy for microcalcifications, several possible explanations should be considered if the pathologist cannot locate the calcifications.

  - Large calcifications may be lost or sheared off as tissue is processed.

  - Calcium oxalate calcifications (associated with fibrocystic lesions) require polarizing microscopy for visualization (malignant calcifications are usually calcium phosphate).

  - The tissue containing the calcifications may not have been sectioned, processed, and looked at. If there is unsectioned tissue, it may be worthwhile doing a specimen radiograph of the unsectioned tissue: the calcifications may be found in the unsubmitted tissue.

  - If all the tissue has been processed, the paraffin blocks can be x-rayed so that the block containing calcifications is identified. This block is then imaged in an orthogonal projection to establish the location (depth) of the calcifications in the block. Calcifications may be deep in the paraffin block, requiring possibly hundreds of slides before the pathologist gets to the calcifications.

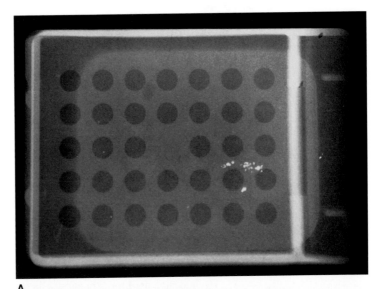

A

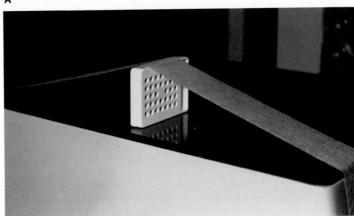

B

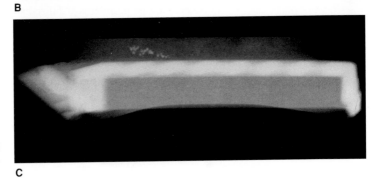

C

FIGURE 14-14
(**A**) Paraffin block containing calcifications. In some patients there are ten to 20 paraffin blocks per biopsy. Isolating the one or two that contain the microcalcifications can be helpful to the pathologist. (**B**) Block oriented vertically and taped to the magnification stand for orthogonal view. (**C**) Orthogonal paraffin block view demonstrating the depth of the calcifications in the block. Many slides would have to be prepared and reviewed before the microcalcifications were reached.

Cyst Aspiration

KEY FACTS

- Indications
  - Symptomatic cysts
  - Atypical features on ultrasound

- Ultrasound
  - Cyst is localized.
  - Using the transducer as a guide, the skin entry site is selected.
  - Can come down directly on cyst—hard to follow needle trajectory and tip; approach used for larger (palpable) cysts
  - Can approach horizontally—needle trajectory can be followed on ultrasound (as done for core biopsy); used for smaller lesions; needle trajectory guided and followed in real time
  - 1% lidocaine used for skin anesthesia (optional)
  - Using a 20G needle, the cyst can be punctured and aspirated.
  - We do not send fluid for cytology unless it is grossly bloody or the patient insists.
  - Most cysts do not need to be aspirated (only if symptomatic or atypical on ultrasound).

- Mammography
  - CC and 90° lateral views are reviewed to establish the shortest skin-to-lesion distance and needle length (see the section above on the parallel to chest wall approach)
  - Using the shortest distance to the lesion, the alphanumeric fenestrated paddle is used to establish the coordinates for the lesion.
  - The needle is advanced slowly as suction is applied. The minute any liquid is obtained, needle position is stabilized and suction is continued until the contents of the cyst have been evacuated completely.
  - Films with the needle still in place are obtained to ensure there is no residual abnormality.
  - If a pneumocystogram is desired (or for therapeutic benefit), air can be injected.

FIGURE 14-15   (A) Lobulated, well-circumscribed mass on mediolateral oblique spot compression view. (B) Complex mass on ultrasound. If aspiration is desired, ultrasound or mammographic guidance can be used. (C) Alphanumeric fenestrated grid used for establishing coordinates of mass (*arrow*) for mammographically guided aspiration. Needle tip is positioned at intersecting point of cross-hairs. Needle is advanced slowly as suction is applied. As soon as fluid is obtained, needle is stabilized and all contents aspirated. Holding the needle steady, needle and syringe are disconnected and an air-filled syringe is connected. Half the aspirated fluid is replaced with air. (D) Pneumocystogram. Smooth-walled, septated cyst. No wall thickening or intracystic abnormality.

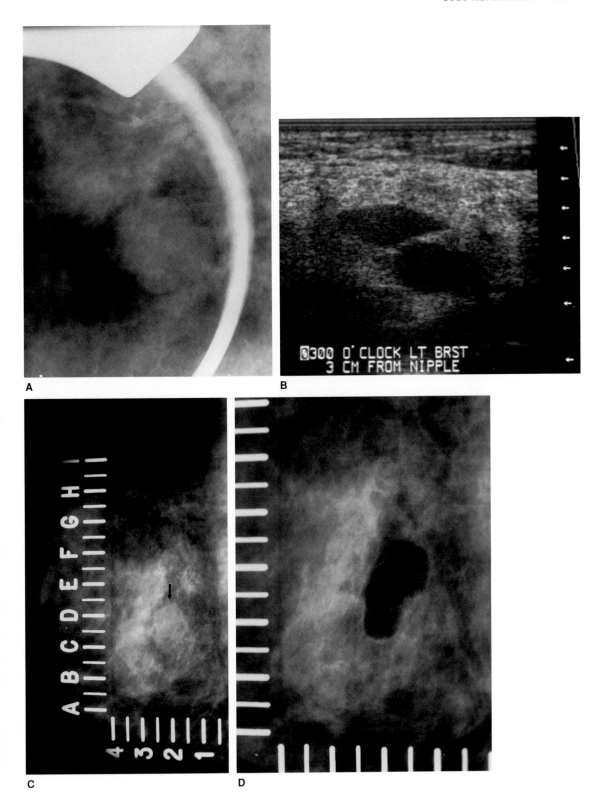

Pneumocystography

KEY FACTS

- Indications
  - Atypical cyst on ultrasound—helps evaluate intracystic or intramural lesions
  - Some have suggested a therapeutic benefit: air may prevent cyst recurrence.
- Procedure
  - After fluid aspiration, 50% of the aspirated fluid is replaced with air.
  - Magnified CC and 90° lateral views are done if evaluation of cyst wall is needed.
  - If air is used for potential therapeutic effect no films are needed.

Ductography

KEY FACTS

GENERAL COMMENTS

- Indication
  - Spontaneous, single-duct nipple discharge

- Clinical
  - Discharge intermittent; patients describe tiny red, brown, to yellowish spots in bra cup or discharge after baths or showers (presumably the hot water relaxes the nipple musculature, facilitating manifestation of discharge)
  - Most women with intraductal lesions have normal breast examinations. Some have an identifiable "trigger point," a point that when compressed reliably elicits discharge.
  - Ductography provides information on the location of lesions within ducts, the number and extent of lesions, and the distribution of the duct within the breast so that minimal-volume breast biopsies can be done, removing the lesions causing discharge and sparing normal surrounding tissue.
  - May avert a biopsy, if fibrocystic changes or duct ectasia is demonstrated

- Mammography
  - Usually normal
  - Occasionally, dilated duct in isolation or within which there are coarse calcifications

- Contraindications (relative)
  - Mastitis, abscess

- Complications
  - Unusual. We have not had any major complications related to ductography, even in patients with a prior history of contrast allergy. Contrast is not injected intravenously or intraarterially, only small amounts of contrast are used, and if needed most of the contrast can be expressed after the procedure.
  - Duct perforation is rare. Patients may describe a sharp pain when perforation occurs and feel a burning sensation as soon as an attempt is made to inject contrast. No long-term sequelae probably result. The patient can be rescheduled for a follow-up study or, if she is willing, the procedure can be tried again after a 20- to 30-minute wait to permit absorption of the extravasated contrast.

- Pitfalls
  - Air bubbles: well-defined, round lucencies that shift in position between views. Care should be exercised when drawing up the contrast to ensure there is no air in the system.
  - Overinjection of contrast may obscure small lesions. It is best to start with small amounts of contrast (0.2 to 0.4 cc), secure the cannula in the duct, and inject additional contrast as needed to opacify the duct.

(text continues on the next page)

Ductography *(Continued)*

- Overinjection may lead to peripheral extravasation; usually the woman complains of burning when extravasation occurs.
- Pseudolesions: uncommon; initial ductogram demonstrates diffuse duct abnormality not confirmed on subsequent (preoperative) studies; cause unknown, postulated to be intraductal debris, possible blood clots, muscular contraction
- Duct perforation is uncommon. When cannulating the duct, do not force or apply significant pressure. If the patient experiences pain, stop and reassess cannula positioning before trying to advance the cannula.

PROCEDURE

- Comfortable patient: supine position; can be done with patient sitting, but may be more cumbersome and cannulation more difficult
- Comfortable radiologist: sitting
- Good lighting (halogen lamp focused on nipple), magnification of nipple surface provided by magnification lenses attached to glasses or safety goggles
- 30G straight, blunt-tipped sialography needle with attached tubing connected to a 3-cc Luer lock syringe and undiluted isothalamate meglumine (Conray 60, Mallinckrodt, St. Louis). Air bubbles should be eliminated from system
  - At the onset, it is important to spend time identifying the secreting duct orifice. On careful inspection of the nipple, the abnormal duct is often slightly patulous and erythematous compared to adjacent duct openings.
  - After inspection of the nipple, elicit a tiny amount of discharge. This is cleared and the process repeated until the orifice has been identified. If too much discharge is elicited, the fluid floods over other duct openings, making isolation of the discharging duct more difficult.
  - When the discharging duct opening is identified, place the tip of the cannula at the opening. Usually the cannula falls into the duct all the way to the hub; do not apply force.
  - If the woman experiences pain during cannulation, stop and reassess the positioning of the cannula. Cannulation should not hurt; in most women it is painless.
  - With the cannula securely in the duct, inject approximately 0.2 to 0.4 cc of contrast and tape the cannula to the nipple using two pieces of paper tape, one at the 3 o'clock position and the second at 9 o'clock.
- Full paddle orthogonal (CC and 90°) magnification views are obtained and reviewed. Because the cannula remains in the duct, additional contrast can be injected as needed. The cannula also helps tamponade the duct so that injected contrast material is not extruded on compression.
- Duct dilatation is not needed; we do not own duct dilators.
- If difficulty is experienced cannulating duct:
  - Place a warm or hot wash towel directly over the nipple for several minutes; this presumably relaxes the nipple musculature.

- Wipe the nipple with an alcohol wipe to clear any keratin plugs partially occluding the duct openings.
- Pull the nipple up gently; this may straighten the subareolar ducts.
- Apply traction to the nipple.

- Preoperative ductography
  - If a lesion is found on the diagnostic ductogram, we do preoperative ductography.
  - 1:1 combination of methylene blue and Conray 60 is used. The methylene blue stains the duct for the surgeon and the Conray 60 permits verification that the abnormal duct has been cannulated.
  - If a lesion is distal to many branch points in the duct or several centimeters from the nipple, needle localization can be done, using the ductogram to direct wire placement.

FINDINGS

- Duct dilatation—as an isolated finding or associated with other findings; obstruction, wall irregularity, expansion and distortion, displacement, or cyst opacification

- Normal ducts
  - Not much has been written on normal duct anatomy, but it probably varies during different physiologic phases of a woman's life.
  - Duct distribution is variable: some ducts diverge to supply large portions of the breast and others terminate close to the nipple with little if any branching.
  - In a few women, opacification of lobules is seen ("lobular blush").

- Solitary papillomas
  - Discharge produced by papillomas can be clear, yellow, brown, or bloody; it is not usually green or white.
  - Solitary papillomas are the most common cause of spontaneous nipple discharge. Approximately 50% of women with spontaneous nipple discharge have solitary papillomas.
  - The papilloma-containing duct is often dilated. Although the dilatation can be diffuse, it most commonly involves the segment of the duct between the papilloma and the nipple.
  - The papilloma itself can produce complete duct obstruction (a meniscus is usually seen), an intraductal filling defect, an intraductal filling defect with expansion and apparent distortion of the duct, or duct wall irregularity (more sessile-like papillomas).
  - With intraductal lesions, biopsy is recommended (cannot distinguish benign from malignant).

- Fibrocystic changes
  - In women with underlying fibrocystic disease, discharge is commonly greenish.

(text continues on next page)

Ductography *(Continued)*

- Opacification of cyst or cysts; duct otherwise normal
- Diffuse duct irregularity—biopsy required (cannot distinguish benign from malignant)
- Duct ectasia
  - Ductal dilatation in the absence of a focal duct abnormality
  - Involved ducts are often attenuated or pruned in appearance.
- Breast cancer
  - Filling defect or defects, abrupt duct cut-off—mass at cut-off site, duct wall irregularity, duct displacement (draping around a lesion)
  - Extravasation—when this occurs because of an underlying duct lesion, the patient does not experience pain during cannulation or burning when contrast is injected. If on your first try you think you might have perforated the duct, bring the woman back and determine if the extravasation occurs again. It is postulated that abnormal ducts may become "leaky," permitting extravasation without perforation.
  - Many of these women have normal physical examinations and mammograms. Generally, the abnormalities on ductography are more extensive with underlying breast cancer than with papillomas. Also, there is less duct distention with malignancy compared with ducts containing solitary central papillomas.

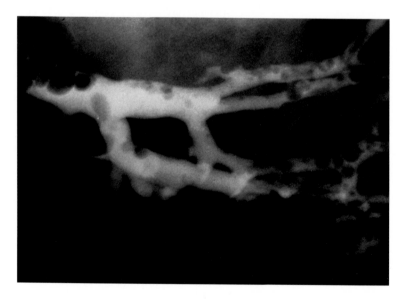

FIGURE 14-16
Air bubbles. Round lucencies throughout duct. Air bubbles shift in position between views.

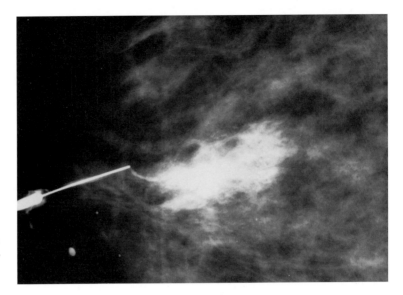

FIGURE 14-17
Hypoplastic duct. Contrast extravasation observed quickly. Patient experiences burning when extravasation occurs.

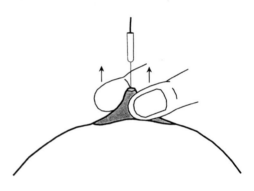

FIGURE 14-18
If there is difficulty cannulating the duct, lifting the nipple as cannulation is attempted can facilitate the needle's falling into the duct.

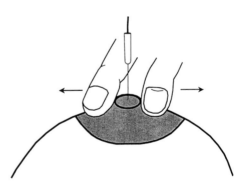

FIGURE 14-19
Tension on the nipple is another maneuver that can be helpful when attempting to cannulate the duct. The tension can help widen duct openings. A warm or hot towel applied directly to the nipple and wiping the nipple clean of keratin plugs are other maneuvers that can be tried during difficult cannulations. In most patients, cannulation is easy and painless.

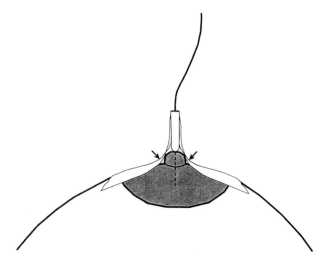

FIGURE 14-20
With the cannula in the duct all the way to the hub, two pieces of paper tape are used to secure it in place. Leaving the cannula in the duct tamponades the duct during compression (contrast is not squeezed back out), and additional contrast can be injected as needed for duct evaluation.

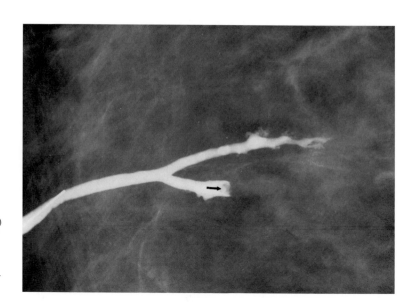

FIGURE 14-21
Complete duct obstruction (*arrow*) by papilloma. Compare caliber of duct to cannula (mild duct dilatation). Because benign and malignant findings overlap on ductography, biopsy is recommended.

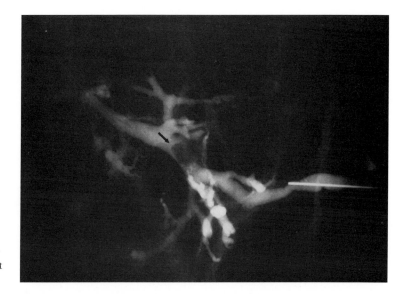

FIGURE 14-22
Filling defect (*arrow*) produced by papilloma. Compare caliber of duct to cannula (mild duct dilatation).

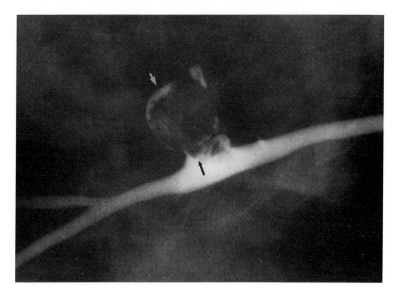

FIGURE 14-23
Papilloma (*black arrow*) appears to be occluding side branch of duct. Some contrast can be seen going around the obstructing lesion (*white arrow*).

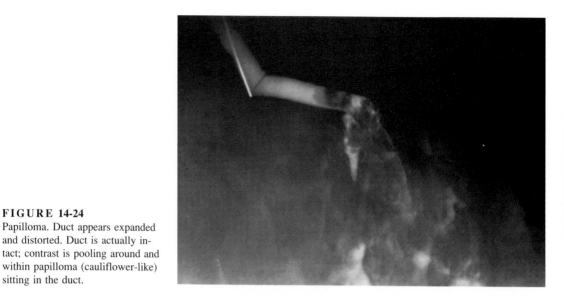

FIGURE 14-24
Papilloma. Duct appears expanded and distorted. Duct is actually intact; contrast is pooling around and within papilloma (cauliflower-like) sitting in the duct.

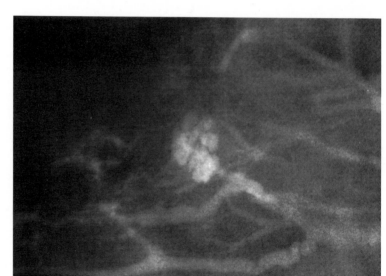

FIGURE 14-25
Opacification of cyst. Lobulated appearance presumably related to incomplete distention of acini.

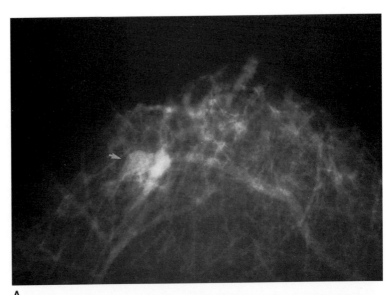

A

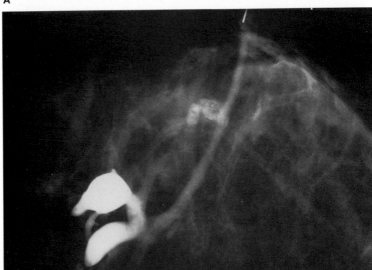

B

FIGURE 14-26

(**A**) Craniocaudal view. Apparent mass (*arrow*) laterally. Patient with spontaneous nipple discharge. (**B**) Opacification of the mass with contrast during ductography. Biopsy can be averted when either cysts or hairpin turns in ducts explain mammographic findings and nipple discharge. Interestingly, discharge often decreases or stops after ductography, for an unknown reason (not extensively documented).

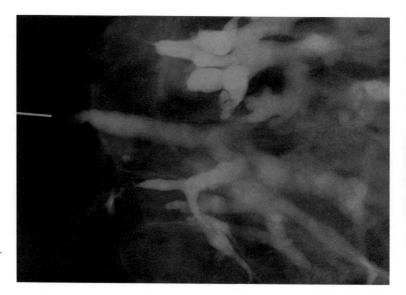

FIGURE 14-27
Duct ectasia. Markedly dilated duct
with no focal duct abnormality identified. In these patients, surgery
may also be averted.

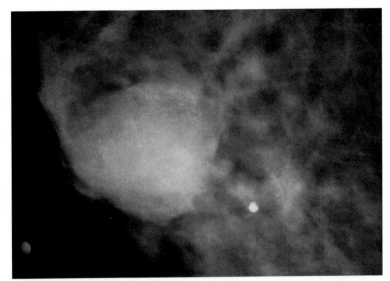

A

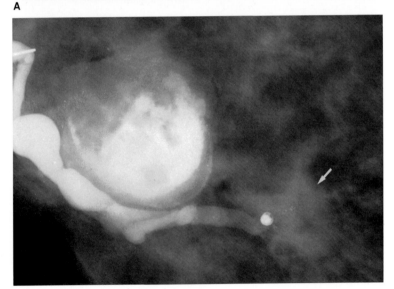

B

FIGURE 14-28
(**A**) Grossly bloody nipple discharge. Mass with ill-defined margins mammographically; no other abnormality detected on the preductogram mammogram. (**B**) Mass seen mammographically is opacified and an irregular filling defect is present. At the time of surgery, when the mass was dissected open, a smooth inner lining was present on gross inspection; the filling defect was an easily removed blood clot. Histologically, this dominant mass was an epithelial-lined cyst. Abrupt duct cut-off with an irregular spiculated mass (*arrow*) surrounding the obstructed duct became apparent on the magnification views done as part of ductography. Punctate calcifications are appreciated in the mass on the magnification views. Histologically, this is an infiltrating ductal carcinoma. Remember: if you find one abnormality, don't stop looking and don't be distracted by the obvious.

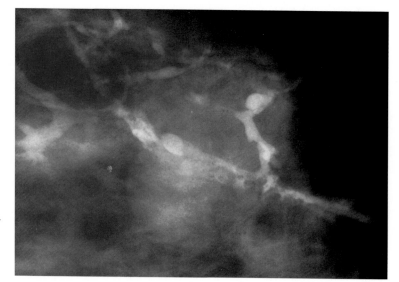

FIGURE 14-29
Patient with bloody nipple discharge, no palpable abnormality, and no associated microcalcifications mammographically. Poorly differentiated ductal carcinoma in situ diffusely involving the opacified duct. The duct is not particularly distended.

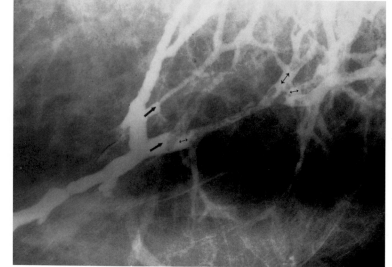

FIGURE 14-30
Spontaneous nipple discharge in patient with no palpable abnormality and no microcalcifications mammographically. Focal areas of duct narrowing (*single and double arrows*) approximately 5 to 7 cm from nipple. Without the ductogram, would the surgeon have dissected back far enough to remove the lesion? Would she or he have known in which direction and how far back to go? Histologically, a ductal carcinoma in situ was diagnosed.

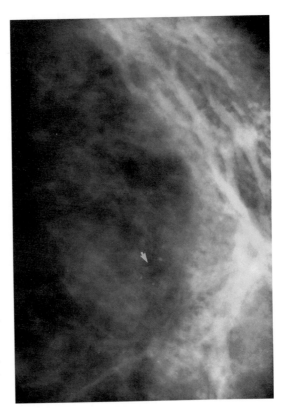

FIGURE 14-31
Spontaneous nipple discharge in a woman with no palpable abnormality and a normal mammogram. Duct displacement (ducts appeared draped over area of tissue containing calcifications) and microcalcifications (*arrow*) on ductography (magnified image). Well- and poorly differentiated (mixed micropapillary, cribriform, comedo) ductal carcinoma in situ with areas of invasion measuring 3.5 cm.

Fine-Needle Aspiration

KEY FACTS

- Aspiration of cellular material from breast lesions for cytologic evaluation
- Guidance
  - Palpation
  - Mammography
  - Ultrasound
  - Stereotactic
- Sterile technique and 1% lidocaine for local anesthesia
- Can use an aspiration device combining a 20-cc syringe with the selected needle or a butterfly needle with a syringe attached to the end of the tubing (this may allow closer control of the needle, particularly during needle excursions—an assistant can apply suction through the attached syringe)
- 22G or 25G needle directed to the center of the lesion
- Needle-tip positioning verified by whichever guidance technology is being used
- Once needle-tip positioning is satisfactory, suction is applied and needle excursions (small, short, quick strokes) varying needle angle are undertaken in the lesion.
- Suction is stopped, the needle is pulled out of the breast, the needle and syringe are separated, air is sucked into the syringe, the needle and syringe are reconnected, and the plunger on the syringe is compressed so that the material in the needle is gently forced out onto a glass slide.
- The edge of a second glass slide is placed on the slide containing the cytologic material at a 45° angle and used to smear the aspirated material.
- Working with the pathologist, these slides can be processed immediately. Drying, fixing, and staining should be in the purview of the pathologist.
- Good results can be obtained using optimal technique and a well-trained, experienced cytopathologist to establish specimen adequacy.

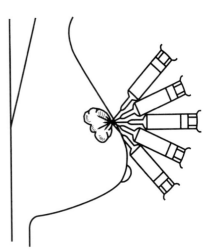

FIGURE 14-32
With the needle in the center of the mass to be sampled, short, quick excursions varying the angle of the needle are undertaken as suction is applied. After sampling, suction is stopped and the needle is withdrawn. It is important to stop suction before pulling the needle out; otherwise, aspirated material may be sucked into the syringe.

Core Biopsy (Stereotactic)

KEY FACTS

- Clinical
    - Core biopsies can be undertaken on most mammographically or ultrasonographically detected breast abnormalities. Caution should be exercised when well-differentiated ductal carcinoma in situ (DCIS), a radial scar/complex sclerosing lesion, or a papillary lesion is suspected: sampling errors may preclude appropriate histologic diagnosis.
    - At many facilities, the use of stereotactic equipment is often limited to women with microcalcifications. Lesions that can be seen on ultrasound are sampled using ultrasound guidance.
    - Given the good results obtained with mammographic or ultrasound guidance, we do not do any needle localizations with the stereotactic unit. Because the breast is compressed in the direction in which the wire is engaged, we actually consider this a relative contraindication: with breast decompression, the final wire position cannot be controlled adequately ("accordion effect").
    - With incongruent radiology/pathology results, atypical ductal hyperplasia, a radial scar/complex sclerosing lesion, possible phyllodes or a papillary lesion on core biopsies, excisional biopsy is recommended.

- Procedure
    - Approach is selected using shortest skin-to-lesion distance (the Fischer unit does not allow an inferior approach).
    - Breast is positioned and a scout view obtained.
    - If the lesion is within the fenestrated portion of the compression paddle, stereo views are obtained.
    - Stereo pair: 15° to the right of midline and 15° to the left of midline
    - Biopsy sites are selected, and using reference points the computer calculates horizontal, vertical, and depth coordinates.
    - 1% lidocaine is used for local anesthesia. Care should be taken not to use too much lidocaine in the breast: the generated blush may obscure a mass, or calcifications in a cluster can be dispersed.
    - Using a #11 surgical blade, a small skin incision is made, large enough for the 14G needle to pass through the skin unimpeded. All passes can usually be made through one skin nick.
    - The needle is advanced through the skin nick to the predetermined depth.
    - Prefire films are obtained to establish the relation of the needle to the lesion (if the needle is on target).
    - The needle is withdrawn approximately 5 mm and fired.
    - Postfire images are obtained to document final needle position.
    - With digital systems, some of the above steps are shortened or may be omitted altogether.
    - The needle is withdrawn and the specimen is teased off the needle into 10% buffered formalin.

- Several passes can be made per lesion (for most lesions an average of four or five passes).
- When the procedure is over, the technologist applies pressure at the biopsy site for 10 minutes.
- An ice pack is placed over the biopsy site and the woman is sent home with the ice pack.
- The patient is provided a telephone number for access to the radiologist should there be complications, questions, or concerns.
- We communicate all biopsy results to patients the next day.
- If the results are benign, the patient is advised when she should have her next mammogram.
- If the results are malignant, the patient's doctor is contacted and surgical referral arranged.
- Relative contraindications
  - Coumadin or aspirin therapy—if coumadin cannot be stopped, tamponade for several minutes after each pass
  - Lesion location—if close to the chest wall, may not be approachable with stereotactic equipment (cannot get the lesion in the window)
  - Patient who cannot lie prone with neck turned for at least 1 hour
  - Some types of lesions (suspected radial scar, well-differentiated DCIS, papillary lesions)

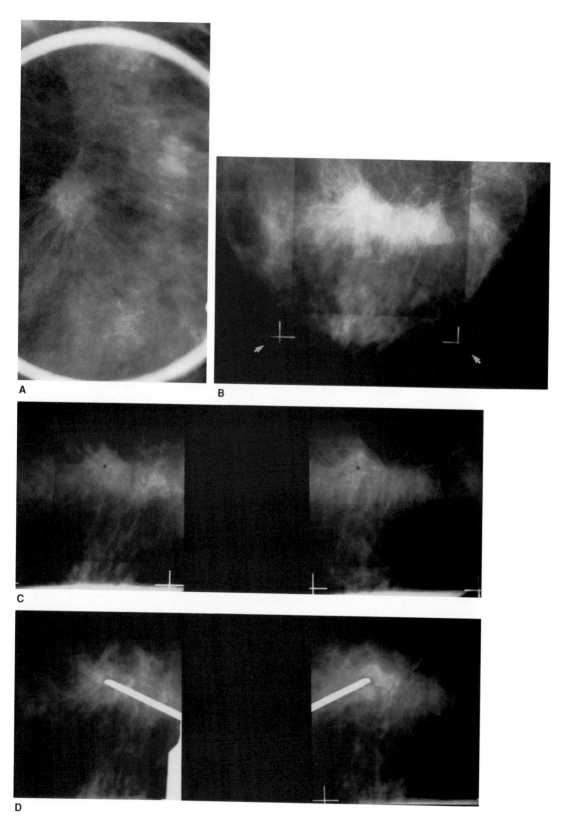

A

B

C

D

FIGURE 14-33   *(See legend on opposite page)*

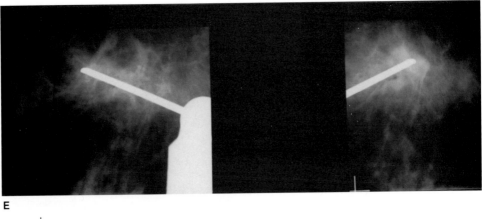

E

F

FIGURE 14-33   (**A**) Micro-focus spot magnification view. Spiculated mass. (**B**) Scout view in craniocaudal projection. Fenestrated window with reference points (*arrows*) on either side of fenestration. With lesion in the window, stereo views are obtained. (**C**) Stereo views. 15° to the right of midline and 15° to the left of midline. Reference points are seen associated with each stereo view. Biopsy sites are selected. In this case, biopsy site through the center of the lesion was selected (dot in center of spiculated mass). Additional biopsies are done at the 12, 3, 6, and 9 o'clock positions. By providing the computer with the reference points and selected biopsy sites, it calculates the depth and vertical and horizontal coordinates. Many of these steps are eliminated and the overall procedure time is reduced with the digital systems now available. (**D**) Prefire stereo views. The needle has been advanced to the computer-generated depth. The needle and the lesion are lined up. Before firing, the needle is withdrawn approximately 0.5 mm. (**E**) Postfire stereo views. After needle firing, stereo views are done to document final needle position. On average, four or five passes are made for masses and suspected poorly differentiated DCIS-type calcifications. The number of passes may be increased (ten to 12 passes) when well-differentiated ductal carcinoma in situ is suspected. Some think this calcification type should be excised rather than subjected to core biopsy. (**F**) After postfire views, the needle is removed from the breast and the inner cannula advanced so that the tissue core can be removed from the tissue slot. The cores are placed in 10% buffered formalin. Fatty specimens float in formalin. Specimens from fibrous or cancerous lesions or hemorrhagic specimens usually sink to the bottom of the formalin canister.

(figure continued on next page)

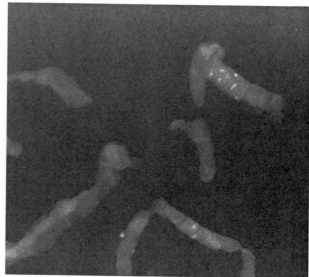

FIGURE 14-33 (CONTINUED)
(**G**) Core radiographs. When stereotactic biopsy of microcalcifications is done, radiographs of the cores can be obtained to verify that calcifications have been removed.

G

Core Biopsy (Ultrasound)

KEY FACTS

- Clinical
  - Most of our core biopsies are done using ultrasound guidance.
  - Easier on the patient (supine position, neck is not turned, no compression) and quicker
  - Must be able to see the lesion well. If there is any question of correlation, leave the anesthesia needle in place and do a mammogram to verify that the mammographically detected lesion and the ultrasound lesion are the same.

- Procedure
  - Lesion localized and approach selected
  - Sterile technique and 1% lidocaine used
  - Skin nick made using #11 surgical blade
  - With the transducer over the lesion (real-time imaging), the needle is advanced, aiming at the midportion of the short transducer axis. Transducer orientation can be used to line the needle up visually with the lesion.
  - Use transducer movements to determine the direction of the needle trajectory.
  - When the needle and lesion are lined up, fire the needle.
  - Needle movement can be assessed in real time.
  - Postfire image is obtained.
  - The needle is withdrawn and the sample teased into 10% buffered formalin.

- This same approach can be used for needle localizations. When the tip of the needle is beyond the lesion, the wire can be engaged.
  - For mammographically visible lesions, the final relation of the wire to the lesion should be verified by obtaining films. These are also helpful in orienting the surgeon to the lesion location. Use a marker (metallic BB) on the skin-entry site for wire.

- Core biopsies are an easier and more practical way of arriving at a diagnosis. They are more cost-effective than surgical biopsies (core biopsies average a third the cost of excisional biopsies), and they leave no scar.

- Core biopsies, however, should not be used to replace or subvert complete diagnostic work-ups of patients with breast-related findings. They should not be used to replace 6-month follow-ups for probably benign lesions.

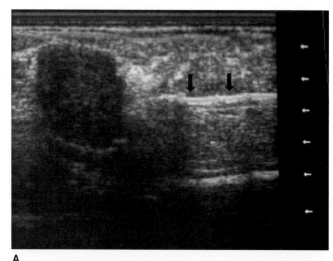

A

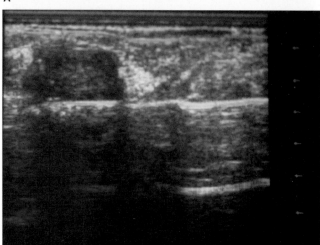

FIGURE 14-34
Ultrasound-guided core biopsy. (**A**) Prefire
view. Needle (*arrows*) lined up with solid hypoechoic mass. Fibroadenoma. (**B**) Postfire view.
Needle has gone through mass. Fibroadenoma.

B

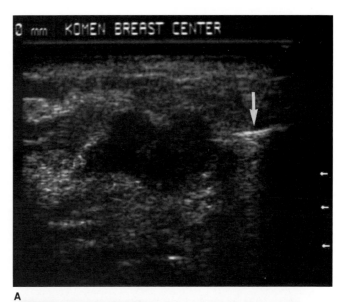

A

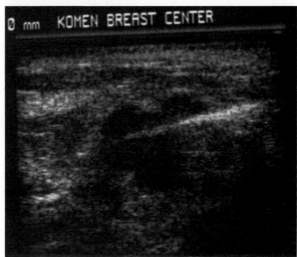

FIGURE 14-35
Ultrasound-guided core biopsy. (**A**) Prefire view. Needle (*arrow*) lined up with irregular, solid hypoechoic mass. Infiltrating ductal carcinoma. (**B**) Postfire view. Needle now seen through the mass. Infiltrating ductal carcinoma.

B

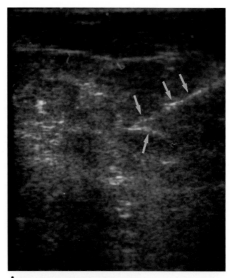

A

FIGURE 14-36

(**A**) Ultrasound-guided needle localization. Needle can be placed through mass under real time, followed by engagement of wire. Occasionally wire hook can be seen in real time, as in this patient. Wire hook is actually within the mass. (**B**) Specimen radiograph documenting lesion removal. Infiltrating ductal carcinoma.

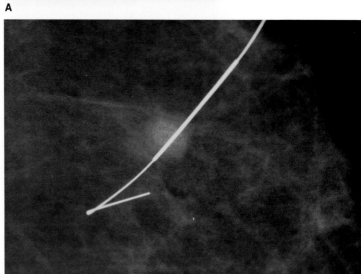

B

Guns and Needles

KEY FACTS

- Needles
    - Inner tissue sampling needle: 4- to 5-mm needle tip followed by a tissue slot (available in different sizes)
    - Outer cutting cannula
    - In prebiopsy position, the outer cannula covers the inner needle.
    - For biopsy, the inner needle is advanced forward (the tip has a downward bevel), and the outer cannula follows immediately, cutting the tissue sample.
    - Different needle lengths: 16 and 10 cm (10 cm commonly used for ultrasound procedures)
- Guns
    - Spring-powered
    - Two sets of springs to move two sections of core biopsy needles
    - Cocking mechanism
    - Safety device
    - Trigger
- "Throw" is the distance traveled by the needle. A short throw (10 to 15 mm) is not recommended because of poor tissue samples; a long throw (21 to 25 mm) is preferred.
- Disposable guns and needles: used for one lesion and then entire mechanism discarded
- Most facilities have reusable guns and disposable needles.

Radiology/Pathology Correlation Sessions

KEY FACTS

- When making a breast biopsy recommendation, consider what you would accept for a diagnosis.

- All breast biopsy results (from excisional and core biopsies) should be reviewed by the radiologists involved. The mammography report, screening and work-up films and studies, specimen radiography, and the pathology report are reviewed.

- Data gathering for medical audit

- Permits determination of radiology/pathology correlation

- If pathology results are incongruent with radiologic impression, more histopathologic review can be undertaken. If needed, the patient can be reevaluated.

  - For example, if you have a dense, solid mass and the pathology report concludes "lipoma," something is wrong. Either the area of radiographic concern was not excised, or it was not included in the material reviewed histologically.

  - If a biopsy was done for microcalcifications and no calcifications are mentioned in the pathology report, you need to go back and establish the whereabouts of the calcifications (presumably seen on specimen radiograph).

- Based on the radiology/pathology reviews, needed follow-ups are established.

  - If the pathology results are not congruent with imaging, immediate evaluation of the patient may be recommended.

  - If there is a high-risk marker lesion, a 6-month follow-up is recommended to establish a new baseline for the patient (see Chap. 12).

  - With core biopsy results indicating atypical ductal hyperplasia, possible radial scar/complex sclerosing lesion, or a papillary lesion, excisional biopsy is usually recommended.

- Learning tool: interpretive abilities can be improved by thorough radiology/pathology reviews.

BIBLIOGRAPHY

Azavedo E, Svane G, Auer G. Stereotactic fine needle biopsy in 2594 mammographically detected nonpalpable lesions. Lancet 1989;1:1033–1035

Cardenosa G, Doudna C, Eklund GW. Ductography of the breast: technique and findings. AJR 1994;162:1081–1087

Cardenosa G, Eklund GW. Paraffin block radiography following breast biopsies: use of orthogonal views. Radiology 1991;180:873–874

Cardenosa G, Eklund GW. Benign papillary neoplasms of the breast: mammographic findings. Radiology 1991;181:751–755

Cardenosa G, Eklund GW. Interventional procedures in breast imaging (parts I & II). In Taveras JM, Ferrucci JT (eds). Radiology. Philadelphia, JB Lippincott, 1993

Czarnecki DJ, Feider HK, Splittgerber GF. Toluidine blue dye as a breast localization marker. AJR 1989;153:261–263

Davis PS, Wechsler RJ, Feig SA, March DE. Migration of breast biopsy localization wire. AJR 1988;150:787–788

Dershaw DD (ed). Interventional breast procedures. New York, Churchill Livingstone, 1996

Fajardo LL, Jackson VP, Hunter TB. Interventional procedures in diseases of the breast: needle biopsy, pneumocystography and galactography. AJR 1992;158:1231–1238

Fornage BD, Coan JD, David CL: Ultrasound-guided needle biopsy of the breast and other interventional procedures. Radiol Clin North Am 1992;30:167–185

Gallagher WJ, Cardenosa G, Rubens JR, et al. Minimal-volume excision of nonpalpable breast lesions. AJR 1989;153:957–961

Gisvold JJ, Martin JK. Prebiopsy localization of nonpalpable breast lesions. AJR 1984;143: 477–481

Hall FM, Frank HA. Preoperative localization of nonpalpable breast lesions. AJR 1979;132: 101–105

Hirsch JI, Banks WL Jr., Sullivan JS, Horsley JS II. Effect of methylene blue on estrogen-receptor activity. Radiology 1989;171:105–107

Holland R. The role of specimen x-ray in the diagnosis of breast cancer. Diagn Imaging Clin Med 1985;54:178–185

Homer MJ. Nonpalpable breast lesion localization using a curved-end retractable wire. Radiology 1985;157:259–260

Homer MJ, Smith TJ, Safaii H. Prebiopsy needle localization. Radiol Clin North Am 1992; 30:139–153

Ikeda DM, Helvie MA, Adler DD, et al. The role of fine-needle aspiration and pneumocystography in the treatment of impalpable breast cysts. AJR 1992;158:1239–1241

Jackson VP. The status of mammographically guided fine needle aspiration biopsy of nonpalpable breast lesions. Radiol Clin North Am 1992;30: 155–166

Kalisher L. An improved needle for localization of nonpalpable breast lesions. Radiology 1978;128:815–817

Kopans DB. The positive predictive value of mammography. AJR 1992;158:521–526

Kopans DB, Deluca S. A modified needle-hookwire breast lesion localizer. AJR 1982;138: 586–587

Kopans DB, Lindfors K, McCarthy KA, Meyer JE. Spring hookwire breast lesion localizer: use of rigid-compression mammographic systems. Radiology 1985;157:537–538

Kopans DB, Meyer J. Versatile spring hookwire breast lesion localizer. AJR 1982;138: 586–587

Kopans DB, Swann CA. Preoperative imaging-guided needle placement and localization of clinically occult breast lesions. AJR 1989;152:1–9

Kopans DB, Waitzkin ED, Linetsky L, et al. Localization of breast lesions identified on only one mammographic view. AJR 1987;149:39–41

Leborgne R. Estudio radiologico del sistema canalicular de la glandula mamaria normal y patologica. Montevideo, Uruguay, Impresora Uruguaya S.A., Juncal 1511, 1943

Leis HP, Cammarata A, LaRaja RD. Nipple discharge: significance and treatment. Breast 1985;11:6–12

Liberman L, Cohen MA, Dershaw DD, et al. Atypical ductal hyperplasia diagnosed at stereotaxic core biopsy of breast lesions: an indication for surgical biopsy. AJR 1995;164: 1111–1113

Liberman L, Evan WP, Dershaw DD, et al. Radiography of microcalcifications in stereotaxic mammary core biopsy specimens. Radiology 1994;190:223–225

Liberman L, Fahs MC, Dershaw DD, et al. Impact of stereotaxic core biopsy on cost of diagnosis. Radiology 1995;195:633–637

Meyer JE. Value of large-core biopsy of occult breast lesions. AJR 1992;158:991–992

Meyer JE, Kopans DB, Stomper PC, Lindfors KK. Occult breast abnormalities: percutaneous preoperative needle localization. Radiology 1984;150:335–337

Parker SH, Burbank F, Jackman RJ, et al. Percutaneous large-core breast biopsy: a multi-institutional study. Radiology 1994;193:359–364

Parker SH, Jobe WE (eds). Percutaneous breast biopsy. New York, Raven Press, 1993

Parker SH, Lovin JD, Jobe WE, et al. Stereotactic breast biopsy with a biopsy gun. Radiology 1990;176:741–747

Parker SH, Lovin JD, Jobe WE, et al. Nonpalpable breast lesions: stereotactic automated large-core biopsies. Radiology 1991;180:403–407

Pollack AH. Localization of breast lesions identified on one mammographic view: the skin-pinch technique. Radiology 1992;185:278–280

Rebner M, Helvie MA, Pennes DR, et al. Paraffin tissue block radiography: adjunct to breast specimen radiography. Radiology 1989;173:695–696

Rebner M, Pennes DR, Baker DE, Adler DD, Boyd P. Two-view specimen radiography in surgical biopsy of nonpalpable breast masses. AJR 1987;149:283–285

Swann CA, Kopans DB, McCarthy KA, et al. Localization of occult breast lesions: practical solutions to problems of triangulation. Radiology 1987;163:577–579

Tabár L, Dean PB. Interventional radiologic procedures in the investigation of lesions of the breast. Radiol Clin North Am 1979;24(3):607–621

Tabár L, Dean PB, Zoltan P. Galactography: the diagnostic procedure of choice for nipple discharge. Radiology 1983;149:31–38

Tabár L, Pentek Z, Dean PB. The diagnostic and therapeutic value of breast cyst puncture and pneumocystography. Radiology 1981;141:659–663

Woods ER, Helvie MA, Ikeda DM, et al. Solitary breast papilloma: comparison of mammographic, galactographic and pathologic findings. AJR 1992;159:487–491

Breast Imaging Companion
by Gilda Cardenosa
Lippincott-Raven Publishers, Philadelphia © 1997

Chapter 15

THE MAMMOGRAPHIC REPORT

General Concepts

KEY FACTS

- Mammography reports should be succinct and accurate.

- For screening studies, two questions must be answered:
    - Is there an area of concern requiring further evaluation?
    - Are there findings consistent with breast cancer?

- For diagnostic studies:
    - Was anything found?
    - What's the next step (eg, return to screening, follow-up, biopsy)?

- Before dictating
    - Review films with comparisons (if available).
    - Decide what you are going to say. Have a clear message, conclusion, and recommendation.
    - Don't use your report to make up your mind or shift responsibility.
    - On clinically occult lesions, the radiologist interpreting the mammogram should provide guidance and a final recommendation. For instance, it makes no sense to say, "Biopsy if clinically indicated" for a cluster of microcalcifications or a nonpalpable mass.

- Read your reports and ask:
    - Do they make sense? Are they logical?
    - Do they reflect accurately what you did?
    - Do you use complete sentences?
    - Do you have run-on sentences?
    - Are your reports helpful to the referring clinician?
    - Get rid of excess verbiage. Every word in your reports should be critical to your message.
    - Your impression should be a conclusion with specific recommendations, not a repeat of what you said in the body of the report.

- Report
    - Type of study (screening, diagnostic, additional views)
    - Tissue type (eg, fatty, fibroglandular, dense)
    - Findings (description), pertinent negatives (if appropriate)
    - Impression
    - Assessment (ACR's *Breast imaging reporting and data system* [BI-RADS] categories—1: negative; 2: benign finding; 3: probably benign finding (short-term follow-up); 4: suspicious abnormality (biopsy should be considered); 5: highly suggestive of malignancy (appropriate action should be taken)

- On all biopsy recommendations, consider making direct contact with the referring physician (document nature of contact and what transpired).

- Consult the ACR's BI-RADS (see bibliography). What follows in this chapter is extracted from this source.

Masses

KEY FACTS

- Shape
  - Round
  - Oval
  - Lobulated, undulations
  - Irregular (when above three terms don't apply)
- Margins
  - Circumscribed—well or sharply defined
  - Microlobulated
  - Obscured—some margins are not well evaluated because of surrounding (potentially superimposed) breast tissue
  - Indistinct—margin definition is poor but not thought to be related to adjacent or superimposed breast tissue
  - Spiculated
- Density
  - X-ray attenuation of mass relative to x-ray attenuation of an equal volume of fibroglandular tissue
  - High density
  - Equal density
  - Low density
  - Fat density
- Location
  - Use clockface preceded by left, right, or bilateral
  - Subareolar, central, or axillary tail
  - Depth (anterior, middle, posterior)
- Associated findings
  - Microcalcifications
  - Architectural distortion
- Size
- Comparison to prior studies
  - How changed

Special Cases

KEY FACTS

- Dilated duct
    - In the absence of other findings (spontaneous nipple discharge), most likely benign
- Intramammary lymph node
    - Fatty hilum
- Asymmetric breast tissue
    - Compared to corresponding area in contralateral breast
    - Different shape on two views
    - In absence of corresponding palpable abnormality, considered benign finding
- Focal asymmetric tissue
    - Similar shape in two views
    - Lacks defined margins of true mass
- Architectural distortion
    - Radiating spicules with no central mass

Calcifications

KEY FACTS

- Benign
    - Skin
    - Vascular
    - Coarse (popcorn-like)
    - Large rod-like (benign ductal—secretory)
    - Round
    - Lucent centered
    - Eggshell or rim
    - Milk of calcium
    - Suture
    - Dystrophic
    - Punctate
- Indeterminate
    - Amorphous or indistinct
- Higher probability of malignancy
    - Pleomorphic or heterogeneous (granular)
    - Linear, branching (casting)
- Distribution
    - Grouped or clustered (small volume, less than 2 cm^3)
    - Linear
    - Segmental
    - Regional (large volume of breast tissue)
    - Diffuse or scattered
- Compared to previous studies
    - How changed

Associated Findings

KEY FACTS

- Can be seen in isolation or associated with masses or calcifications
- Skin or nipple retraction
- Skin thickening
  - Diffuse
  - Focal
- Trabecular thickening
- Axillary adenopathy
- Architectural distortion

BIBLIOGRAPHY

American College of Radiology. Breast imaging reporting and data system (BI-RADS), 2d ed. Reston, VA: ACR, 1995

D'Orsi CJ. Use of the American College of Radiology breast imaging and data system. RSNA Categorical Course in Breast Imaging Syllabus 1995, pp 77–80

D'Orsi CJ, Kopans DB. Mammographic feature analysis. Semin Roentgenol 1993;28: 204–230

Breast Imaging Companion
by Gilda Cardenosa
Lippincott-Raven Publishers, Philadelphia © 1997

Chapter 16

MAMMOGRAPHY AUDIT

General Concepts

KEY FACTS

- Data collection and analysis are aimed at evaluating the accuracy of mammography and mammographic interpretation.

- What are we trying to accomplish by screening women for breast cancer with mammography, and why?
  - Early breast cancer detection can lead to decreases in breast cancer mortality rates.
  - Cancer detection rate and sensitivity: mammography must demonstrate, and we need to detect, a large enough percentage of the breast cancers existing in the population
  - Rate of minimal, node-negative, and node-positive breast cancers detected: the effectiveness of mammography is related to early detection and good prognostic characteristics for the detected breast cancers

- What does it take to detect breast cancer with mammography?
  - Amount of imaging required—recall rates (in finding breast cancers, the number of callbacks and additional imaging studies done should be minimized)
  - How many biopsies for mammographically detected, clinically occult lesions are recommended (versus biopsies done) per breast cancer detected. The positive predictive value (PPV) of breast biopsy recommendations is the number of biopsies recommended (versus biopsies actually done) relative to the number of cancers found.

- Raw data
  - Patient demographics (age, breast cancer history, hormone replacement, previous biopsy-proven high-risk lesions [atypical ductal hyperplasia, lobular neoplasia/lobular carcinoma in situ])
  - Audit period dates
  - Number of screening and diagnostic studies
  - Number of recalls
  - Number of excisional biopsy recommendations (fine-needle aspirations and core biopsies tracked separately)
  - Biopsy results
  - Tumor staging
  - Number of first-time screens
  - Number of repeat screens

- Derived data
  - Number of true-positive (TP), false-positive (FP), false-negative (FN), and true-negative (TN) results
  - PPV
  - Cancer detection rate
  - Percentage of minimal breast cancers detected

- • Percentage of node-positive breast cancers detected
- • Recall rate
- • Prevalent versus incident breast cancer rates

• When reviewing reports on audit results, be sure that what was done and calculated is defined precisely: some of these terms are defined differently by different investigators.

Definitions

KEY FACTS

- TP
  - Breast cancer diagnosed within 1 year after biopsy recommendation for an abnormality detected on mammography

- TN
  - No breast cancer diagnosed within 1 year of a normal mammogram

- FN
  - Breast cancer detected within 1 year of a normal mammogram
  - Probably the least accessible number in an audit. If patients move out of the area or are managed at another institution, the finding of breast cancer may not be communicated to the original institution.
  - Affects the TN

- FP—several definitions, so be sure this is defined specifically
  - FP1—no breast cancer diagnosed within 1 year of a recall or biopsy recommendation
  - FP2—no breast cancer diagnosed within 1 year following a biopsy recommendation for an abnormal mammogram
  - FP3—biopsy with benign findings within 1 year of a biopsy recommendation based on an abnormal mammogram

- Sensitivity
  - Probability of detecting breast cancer when cancer is present (TP/[TP + FN]); how good is mammography at detecting breast cancer?

- Specificity
  - Probability of a normal mammogram when no breast cancer exists (TN/[FP + TN]); how good is the test at determining the absence of disease?
  - Varies depending on which definition of FP is used; the variation, however, is not significant because TN is usually a much larger number than FP

- PPV—several definitions depending on what is being looked at

- PPV of abnormal findings at screening (PPV 1): percentage of screening studies with abnormal findings that result in a diagnosis of breast cancer (TP/[TP + FP1])

- PPV of biopsy recommendations (PPV 2): percentage of patients recommended for biopsy that resulted in a diagnosis of breast cancer (TP/[TP + FP2])

- PPV of biopsies done (PPV 3): percentage of all known biopsies done that resulted in a diagnosis of breast cancer (TP/[TP + FP3])

- Breast cancer detection rate

- Number of breast cancers found per 1000 patients examined with mammography

- Minimal breast cancer
  - Invasive carcinomas 1 cm or less or ductal carcinoma in situ

- Interval breast cancers
  - Breast cancers becoming clinically apparent following a negative mammogram and before the next screening mammogram

Goals

KEY FACTS

- Sensitivity of mammography
  - Should exceed 85%
  - Hard to calculate because in most practice settings, an accurate FN rate is difficult to obtain
- PPV
  - Related directly to ages in the population being screened
  - Usually varies directly with tumor size being found
  - Varies depending on the definition of PPV used
  - Nationally, PPV 2 = 21%
  - Range, 25% to 40%
  - For screening facilities, PPV 1 should be used: 5% to 10%
- Tumor size
  - Varies depending on ratio of screening to diagnostic studies
  - More than 50% of tumors diagnosed by mammography are stage 0 or 1.
  - More than 30% of mammographically detected breast cancers are minimal.
- Node-positive breast cancers
  - Tumor size correlated with node positivity
  - Less than 25% of screen-detected breast cancers should be node-positive.
- Cancer detection rate
  - Varies depending on prevalence versus incidence
  - Varies depending on age of population being screened, as breast cancer increases in incidence with age
  - Six to ten cancers/1000 women screened—among first-time screens: prevalent cancer rate
  - Two to four cancers/1000 women screened—among repeat screens: incident cancer rate
- Recall rate
  - May decrease directly with experience of mammographer
  - Varies depending on number of first-time screens versus repeat screens
  - Cost-effectiveness and credibility of mammography will be questioned if recall rate is too high.
  - 10% or less has been reported.
- Specificity
  - Must know all TN results, which in turn requires knowledge of FN results (least accessible number in audit)
  - More than 90%

Benefits of Auditing

KEY FACTS

- Measuring the success of a mammography program and that of each mammographer in finding breast cancer
- Teaching and learning tool
- Identification of FN studies—review of FN results may lead to an understanding of how these can be avoided in the future—continuous quality improvement
- Outcome analysis can be used at local and national levels.
- If benefit is demonstrated, may improve compliance of referring physicians and patients
- Calculation of costs per patient screened
- Medicolegal: a radiologist's profile may be helpful in demonstrating the appropriateness of the steps taken (eg, follow-up of lesions with a low likelihood of malignancy versus biopsy)

BIBLIOGRAPHY

Linver MN, Osuch JR, Brenner RJ, Smith RA. The mammography audit: a primer for the Mammography Quality Standards Act (MQSA). AJR 1995;165:19–25

Sickles EA. Quality assurance: how to audit your own mammography practice. Radiol Clin North Am 1992;30:265–275

Sickles EA. Auditing your practice. RSNA Syllabus Categorical Course in Breast Imaging 1995, pp 81–91

Breast Imaging Companion
by Gilda Cardenosa
Lippincott-Raven Publishers, Philadelphia © 1997

Chapter 17

EMERGING TECHNOLOGIES

Magnetic Resonance Imaging

KEY FACTS

- Potential indications
  - Extent of disease—multifocal disease
  - Staging of breast cancer
  - Implant evaluation—can detect gel bleed and intracapsular rupture
  - Recurrence (versus scar tissue) after lumpectomy and radiation therapy
  - Evaluation of dense breast tissue
- Development of biopsy techniques for magnetic resonance-detected lesions (clinically and mammographically occult) is ongoing.

Digital

KEY FACTS

- Already in use for localization and core biopsy (using small field of view)
    - Shortens procedure time by eliminating film processing
- Permits image manipulation, potentially improving depiction of breast cancers
- Detection and analysis
    - Charge-coupled device—current field of view limited, precludes full field; resolution of 8 line pair/mm compared with 13 to 15 for current mammography x-ray systems
    - Scanning with small CCd
        - Increased dose
        - Prolonged exposure times (with resultant blurring)
        - X-ray tube overload
    - Photostimulable phosphors—can image whole breast; resolution limited; resolution of 1 to 5 line pair/mm
    - Digitization of standard mammogram

Computer-Aided Diagnosis

KEY FACTS

- Digitized images
- Computer programs (actively under development) to detect microcalcifications, masses, and architectural distortion on digitized images
- Intended to improve the radiologist's detection performance
- Must deal with false-positive results (the computer marking every minute or benign microcalcification [eg, vascular]); must reduce false-positive rate while maintaining high sensitivity
  - Also to be determined: appropriate specificity

Scintigraphy

KEY FACTS

- Thallium-201 has been used, but all lesions studied were palpable and none smaller than 1.3 cm.

- Technetium-99m sestamibi under investigation

  - Unclear if benign from malignant lesions will be distinguished adequately (potentially eliminating some of the interventional procedures undertaken)

  - Size of lesion detection also a factor; may not reliably identify lesions less than 1.2 cm

  - Uptake related to neovascularity

  - Some cellular uptake also appears to occur (into mitochondria).

Positron Emission Tomography

KEY FACTS

- Benign versus malignant
    - Lesion size a factor; unclear if this method identifies smaller lesions reliably and consistently
- Metabolism
    - Biologically active labeled molecules: glucose labeled with fluorine-18
    - Can we gain prognostic information?
- Presence of axillary nodal metastases

BIBLIOGRAPHY

Davis PL (ed). Breast imaging. MRI Clin North Am, November 1994

Kopans DB. Other breast imaging techniques. RSNA Categorical Course in Breast Imaging Syllabus 1995, pp 209–215

Schmitt RA, Wolverton DE, Vyborny CJ. Computer-aided diagnosis in mammography. RSNA Categorical Course in Breast Imaging Syllabus 1995, pp 199–208

GENERAL READING

American College of Radiology. 1994. ACR standard for diagnostic mammography and problem solving breast evaluation. Reston, VA: author.

American College of Radiology. 1995. ACR standard for screening mammography. Reston, VA: author.

American College of Radiology. Breast imaging reporting and data system (BI-RADS), 2d ed. Reston, Va., American College or Radiology, 1995

Bassett LW (ed). Breast imaging: current status and future directions. Radiol Clin North Am, January 1992

Bassett LW, Hendrick RE, Bassford TL, et al. High-quality mammography: information for referring providers. Quick reference guide for clinicians no. 13. AHCPR Publication No. 95-0633. Rockville, MD, Agency for Health Care Policy and Research, Public Health Service, U.S. Department of Health and Human Services. 1994.

Bassett LW, Hendrick RE, Bassford TL, et al. Quality determinants of mammography. Clinical practice guideline no. 13. AHCPR Publication No. 95-0632. Rockville, MD, Agency for Health Care Policy and Research, Public Health Service, U.S. Department of Health and Human Services. 1994.

Bassett LW, Jackson VP, Jahan R., Fu YS, Gold RH. Diagnosis of diseases of the breast. Philadelphia, Saunders, 1997.

Dershaw DD (ed). Interventional breast procedures. New York, Churchill Livingstone, 1996

Parker SH, Jobe WE (eds). Percutaneous breast biopsy. New York, Raven Press, 1993

Powell DE, Stelling CB. The diagnosis and detection of breast disease. St. Louis, Mosby, 1994

Tabàr L, Dean P. Teaching atlas of mammography. New York, Thieme-Stratton, 1985 (highly recommended)

General Breast Books

Bland KI, Copeland EM (eds). The breast. Philadelphia, WB Saunders, 1991

Haagensen CD. Diseases of the breast, 3d ed. Philadelphia, WB Saunders, 1986

Harris JR, Lippman ME, Morrow M, Hellman S. Diseases of the breast. Philadelphia, Lippincott-Raven, 1996.

Breast Pathology

Azzopardi JG. Problems in breast pathology. London, WB Saunders, 1979

Barth V, Prechtel K. Atlas of breast disease. Philadelphia, BC Decker, 1991

Fechner RD, Mills SE. Breast pathology: benign proliferations, atypias and in-situ carcinomas. Chicago, American Society of Clinical Pathologists, 1990

Page DL, Anderson TJ (eds). Diagnostic histopathology of the breast. New York, Churchill Livingstone, 1987

Tavassoli FA. Pathology of the breast. New York, Elsevier, 1992

INDEX

Page numbers followed by *f* indicate figures.